# Baby Massage

# Baby Massage

## FOR THE VTCT CERTIFICATE

Carole Nyssen

www.heinemann.co.uk
✓ Free online support
✓ Useful weblinks
✓ 24 hour online ordering

**01865 888058**

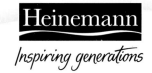

Heinemann Educational Publishers
Halley Court, Jordan Hill, Oxford OX2 8EJ
Part of Harcourt Education

Heinemann is the registered trademark of
Harcourt Education Limited

© Carole Nyssen, 2003

First published 2003

08 07 06 05 04 03
10 9 8 7 6 5 4 3 2 1

British Library Cataloguing in Publication Data is available
from the British Library on request.

ISBN 0 435 45648 2

Designed by Carolyn Gibson
Typeset by J&L Composition, Filey, North Yorkshire
Original illustrations © Harcourt Education Limited, 2003
Illustrated by Jane Bottomley and Kamae Design
Printed in the UK by Bath Press Ltd

### *Acknowledgements*
Every effort has been made to contact copyright holders of material
reproduced in this book. Any omissions will be rectified in
subsequent printings if notice is given to the publishers.

We would like to thank the Vocational Training Charitable Trust
(VTCT) and Heather Mole for their helpful comments in reading
through the book.

The author and publisher would like to thank the following individuals
and organizations for permission to reproduce photographs:
Alamy page 9, 26 (bottom), 51; Gareth Boden page 5; Bubbles pages
17, 20 (top), 26 (top) and 80; Robert Noah Calvert/Massage Mag page
3; Gerald Sunderland page 18–9, 20 (bottom), 21–5, 27–9 and 117
and Bryony J Wilson pages 1, 59, 107 and 123.

# Inspired by and dedicated to Christian and Rachael

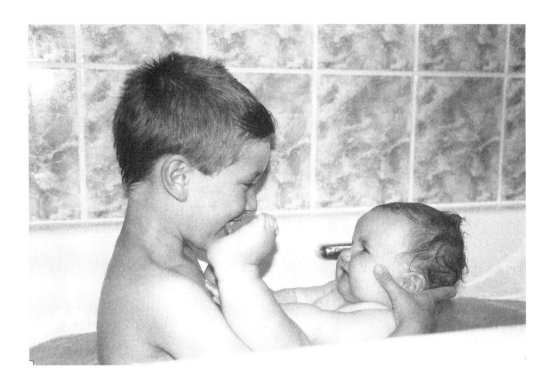

# Contents

# Introduction

Human touch is a natural part of caring. Babies and young children depend on physical contact, and it is often instinctive for carers to communicate and bond with their child through physical touch. Children who are distressed or in pain can be comforted by gently stroking the afflicted area, perhaps rocking the child or speaking quietly to them until they become calm and the pain is gone. Massage can be thought of as a formalised and improved version of these bonding and soothing processes.

The reason for these instincts is clear: massage has crucial benefits. This has been backed up by extensive research into the importance of touch in human development. This research has concluded that children who are touched or massaged from birth develop more quickly in terms of psychological and physical strength and health.

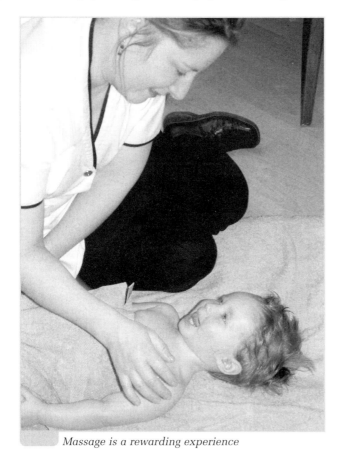

*Massage is a rewarding experience*

The psychological benefits can be seen in the fact that children who grow up without loving care and touch often display behavioural disorders and emotional problems, which stay with them throughout their adult life. There is a strong related socio-psychological benefit: baby massage can lead to a strengthening of the relationship between carer and child. This may be particularly good for fathers, who are able, through massage, to take a more active role in caring for the newborn. In this way massage can become a wonderful and rewarding experience involving the whole family.

The physical benefits of baby massage are even more numerous and immediate than the psychological ones. The benefits range from accelerated growth of the skeleton, muscles and lungs, to the boosting of the immune system, aiding of digestion and simple relaxation! They can counter various infant complaints, or just provide a general physical boost. Massage is very useful, for example, for premature babies since it helps them develop much more quickly than their counterparts.

The Vocational Training and Charitable Trust (VTCT) Baby Massage qualification enables students to perform and teach massage to parents, carers, midwives and health visitors, whilst experiencing for themselves the pleasure of learning a unique discipline that will never be forgotten.

This book contains everything the student needs to support each element of the qualification, which are referenced under Qualification cross-referencing (see page 139). Included at the back of the book are assessment questions and documentation that can be used by the student to form part of their portfolio of evidence.

## The History of Massage

The presence of massage can be dated back as far as the prehistoric age. It is known to be one of the oldest accepted methods in the healing arts to be used by man in the attempt to relieve pain. In many cultures, such as India, Pakistan and some African and West Indian cultures, baby massage is a traditional way of handling children. From birth they are massaged by their mothers, grandmothers and sometimes the midwife, and it becomes part of their daily routine. It is now becoming increasingly recognised in Western civilisation as a part of childcare because of the many benefits it offers.

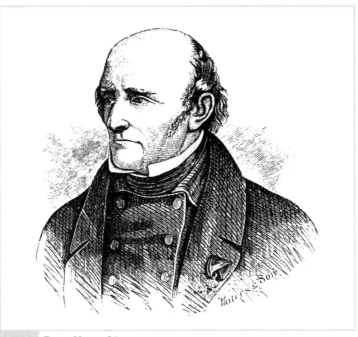
*Peter Henry Ling*

Peter Henry Ling of Sweden (1776–1839) made the most dramatic contribution to massage as we know it today. Ling devoted many years to studying massage in its various forms. From his research he systematically organised the techniques and introduced such terms as **effleurage**, **petrissage**, **friction** and **vibration** (see Classification of massage movements, page 75). Although Ling did not have a medical background he realised the importance of achieving a good understanding of anatomy and physiology before administering massage. He treated only conditions considered to be 'normal', and anything outside of this he quickly recommended to a doctor. The techniques that Ling used and taught have become known as the 'Swedish system' of massage. Yet, masseurs often use French words to describe Swedish massage techniques. This is because French missionaries were the first to describe the classical-type massage techniques. The French names and descriptions quickly became part of the vocabulary for masseurs throughout Europe.

# PART ONE:
# Underpinning knowledge

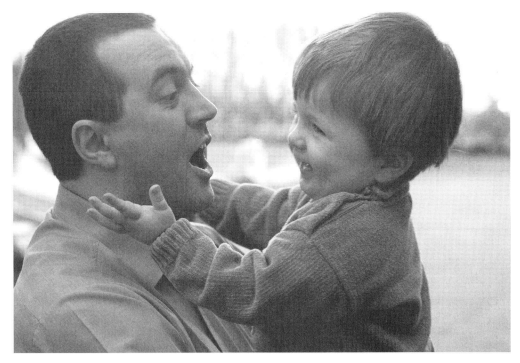

# Professional Practice

## Professional Ethics/Code of Practice

Why do we have a code of practice or professional ethics – what are they for, how do they help us? These questions have been frequently asked by students. All professional working bodies (for example: therapists, nurses, doctors, social workers and health visitors) set their own codes and practices. Codes of practice and ethics are designed to encourage integrity and responsibility within the profession, and to ensure that all members work to similar exacting and uncompromising standards. Ethics are defined as being 'moral principles' or 'rules of conduct'. Codes of practice and ethics are usually outlined by professional organisations and all examining bodies. Practitioners should ensure that they are familiar with those guidelines identified by the organisations of which they are members.

In the case of baby massage more than one set of codes and ethics applies and a practitioner should be aware of their areas of responsibility:

- Always recognise the responsibility that you have towards a parent/guardian and baby. A baby's welfare and comfort should take priority at all times.
- Show sensitivity, tact and discretion at all times when dealing with carers.
- Respect the unique nature of the individual regardless of their race, colour, creed or sex.
- You may refuse to give a massage providing a refusal is carried out in a professional manner. This is relevant in the case of a baby having a **contra-indication** (see Contra-indications to baby massage, page 51) to massage.
- Do not seek to attract business unfairly or unprofessionally or in any way which would discredit the reputation of other therapists. (For example: if a health visitor has an established practice in a particular area of town, you should not attempt to set up the same business in the same area of town – unless of course you can demonstrate a need for the additional practice! Of course if you can do this you must be careful not to discredit the other

practitioner in any way; this a part of the code of practice you share.)

- All advertisements should be accurate, discreet and dignified in tone. You cannot advertise yourself as a baby masseur until you have qualified, and then you cannot claim that massage will solve sleep problems with babies – it doesn't work with all babies!

- Restrict conversation with a carer to impersonal and non-controversial topics. Never inflict opinions on a carer or discuss their private lives! That is not to say you can't make gentle suggestions if a carer is open to ideas. This is something that you will learn to judge for yourself.

- Keep clear and comprehensive records of treatments undertaken, including dates and advice given. This is probably one of the easiest things to get right, and yet so often records are misplaced, incomplete or simply lost. If you went to your doctor for a repeat prescription you would be pretty angry if you couldn't get it because the doctor had 'mislaid' your records, wouldn't you? So, if a carer you saw six months ago returns to you with the same baby and asks you about previous massages, and you don't have the records – what are you going to do?

- You MUST be adequately insured to practise. Freelance workers are probably the most vulnerable to insurance claims.
  (For example, a freelancer recalls an incident when she was freelancing: "I knocked over a bottle of extra-virgin olive oil onto a client's carpet. As hard as we tried we couldn't get it all out and my insurance ended up paying for a new carpet." So be careful, it can happen to anyone!)

- Display professional membership badges and certificates denoting qualifications, etc. to denote professional status and inspire confidence and respect in carers.

- Ensure your ongoing personal professional development by maintaining and updating your training and endeavouring to increase your knowledge.

- Always maintain client confidentiality, which goes for babies as well as their carers.

- Make sure that carers are fully informed about massage procedures.

- Ensure that the carer is present at all times during a massage. Unfortunately, in today's society practitioners have to safeguard themselves against certain possible allegations, particularly where children are involved.

Putting these points into practice ensures that you will work in a professional and safe environment, that keeps your 'client's' best interests at heart.

# Medical Ethics

Like professional ethics and the code of conduct, medical ethics ensure 'good practice'. Most practitioners of baby massage will not be qualified to diagnose, however tempting it is! (If a client's baby is covered in eczema, for example, although most therapists and carers would be familiar with the condition, you should not tell the client what you think it is. Instead you should suggest that a visit to the doctor would be a good idea to get the condition diagnosed.) The diagnosis of any condition lies within the province of the medical profession as does the treatment of that condition. Do not use titles or descriptions to give the impression of having a medical or other qualification, unless you possess them, and make it clear to clients that you are not a doctor and do not have a doctor's knowledge or skill. Once a condition has been diagnosed and treatment has been prescribed, never countermand instructions or prescriptions given by a doctor or undermine a doctor's decision or recommendations.

**SAFE PRACTICE**

*Never allow a baby to undergo treatment if they have a medical condition which contra-indicates it even if the client insists.*

reflect

Work with a partner to see if you can remember six points of professional ethics, and then list six of medical ethics.

# Legislation

Every workplace in the country is governed by legislation and law set down by Acts of Parliament. These are to ensure protection in the health, safety and hygiene of employers, employees and visitors to the workplace. Establishment rules are drawn from the complexities of these acts to ensure standards are met. Failure to comply can lead to very serious consequences and may result in any one of the following:

- **claims for damages from injured staff.** We read in the newspapers every day about claims against companies for injury to their staff, and how it costs the insurance business millions of pounds every year. If running a business, make sure you follow strict health and safety guidelines to

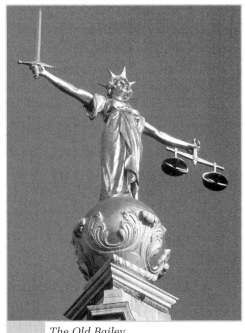

*The Old Bailey*

ensure your staff are protected from possible injury.

- **claims for damages from injured clients.** Many clients have ended up making claims against establishments, and although rare in the baby massage world, it doesn't mean it couldn't happen. To take an example from the world of hairdressing and beauty: a client slipped in the reception area of a salon on a couple of drops of oil. She fell into the display cabinet, scarring her face and breaking her arm at the same time. A freak accident perhaps, but the claim was high because the oil had been spilt over an hour before the incident and hadn't been cleaned up, and because the cabinet the client fell into didn't contain safety glass, which could possibly have withstood the fall. The client won the case. This incident demonstrates how easy it is to fall outside of good working practices and end up with a substantial bill for damages.
- **loss of trade through bad publicity and a damaged reputation.** The family of the injured woman in the example above attracted huge local media attention, which resulted in prosecution and fines and, finally, the closure of the 'offending' business.

The two acts which directly affect the provision of baby massage are outlined below.

## The Local Government (Miscellaneous Provisions) Act 1982 / Local authority by-laws

Precise by-laws vary from one authority to another, but the main focus of the act is on efficient hygiene practices. The safe practice of baby massage is dependent on the following guidelines (babies are so susceptible to germs, infection and cross-infection that it is essential to follow these simple guidelines). The by-laws are made by the local authority to ensure:

- cleanliness of the premises and fittings
- cleanliness and hygiene of the person registered and any assistants
- the sterilisation and disinfecting of instruments, materials and equipment used.

Because of the variations in local legislation it is wise to seek advice from your local authority environmental officer. In authorities where licensing and registration are required it is important to remember that those working from home or who run a visiting practice are still required to register and are subject to inspection. The only exception is for those who are working under medical control, i.e. in a hospital.

If safe hygienic practices are not maintained, the local environmental health officers have the right to fine or cancel registration of a business.

## The Health and Safety at Work Act 1974

The act provides a comprehensive legal framework to promote and encourage high standards of health and safety in the workplace.

Both employer and employee have responsibilities under the act:

| THE EMPLOYER'S DUTY IS TO PROVIDE: | THE EMPLOYEE'S RESPONSIBILITIES ARE TO: |
| --- | --- |
| safe premises, with access to exits | avoid personal injury |
| systems and equipment | assist the employee in meeting the health and safety requirements |
| storage and transport of substances and materials | avoid injury or danger to clients |
| good practices | not misuse or alter anything that has been provided for safety |
| information on health & safety to employees | |
| adequate ventilation, correct working temperature, appropriate lighting, client privacy and low noise levels | |
| protection of employees from health and safety risks | |

The legislation was updated, widening the scope of the existing act. There are now four main areas:

- **manual handling operations;** there are very strict rules about lifting and carrying to protect people from injury in a work situation. This is particularly relevant if you are freelancing; remember, it is better to make two safe trips, than one that ends in injury.
- **provision and use of work equipment;** all equipment provided for you by an employer should be 'Pat' tested on a regular basis. If it is electrical, it should be in good working order and you should have access to instructions on how to use it.
- **workplace health, safety and welfare;** your employer has a responsibility to ensure that you are working in a place that addresses your health, safety and welfare. This includes the requirement that there is adequate light, sufficient heating, toilet facilities and running hot and cold water. Health and safety notices should be visible to all staff, clearly stating what may or may not be done, and what should be done in an emergency.
- **personal protective equipment at work;** PPE for short! If you need to wear rubber gloves for disposing of a nappy, then your employer must provide them for you. Baby massage requires a plastic disposable apron, disposable gloves, paper and an antibacterial soap.

## RIDDOR (Reporting of Injuries, Diseases & Dangerous Occurrences Regulations)

This is part of the Health & Safety at Work Act. No matter how minor, or how serious, legislation requires **all** accidents or injuries to be formally reported. Usually this is in the form of an 'Accident Book' or 'Register'. Included in the legislation is the requirement to report if any employee is off sick for more than three days as a result of an accident at work, or if they have a specified occupational injury or disease that has been certificated by a doctor. For example, the employer of a therapist, suffering from repetitive strain injury (RSI) as a result of many years of massaging, is required to report the injury and ensure the injury is not made worse from the work he or she is doing.

The Local Authority Environmental Health Department requires a report to be sent to them within seven days of the incident. The report should contain the following information:

- details of the person injured, including his or her name, age, gender and address
- details of all persons involved, any witnesses and the person/s who dealt with the situation
- date and place where it happened
- how the accident occurred
- what action was taken, e.g. was the person taken to hospital, home or returned to work?

## The Children Act (1989)

The Children Act (1989) brings together many different pieces of legislation and is based on the idea that, like adults, children have rights. It aims to protect all children but also looks specifically at the needs and rights of vulnerable children. The Act covers issues such as child protection, registration of childcare settings and parental responsibility.

As baby massage involves working directly with babies and children, it is important to be aware of young peoples' rights and how you can support them through your practice. For example, it is essential to have parental consent **prior** to proceeding with the massage, particularly as baby massage involves undressing the baby or child. Indeed, the consent of the baby or child should also be apparent, i.e. never force a child to have massage if they are uncomfortable or irritable.

A full copy of the Act can be found at *www.hmso.gov.uk/acts/* but the key proposals are as follows:

- the welfare of the child must at all times be considered 'paramount'
- children should be consulted and kept informed about decisions that affect their future
- wherever possible, children should be brought up and cared for within their own families
- parents with 'children in need' should be helped to bring up their children themselves.

## Data Protection Act (1998)

Any establishment that stores personal data must be registered under this Act. The Act states that customers / clients have the right to:

- be informed where the data is being processed
- a description of the details being held
- the reason why the data is being processed
- know to whom the data may be disclosed.

As a general rule, sensitive information such as details on race or ethnic origin, health or medical conditions may not be recorded unless the child's parents/carers have given consent. The data can be used only for the purpose for which it was collected. For example, if you collect information about a baby for massage and record it on your consultation log, you cannot then pass that information onto a baby food company. Apart from breaking the law, this would also be unethical!

# Maintaining Employment Standards for the Therapist

Appearance should be considered and hygienic practices maintained at all times in order to protect both the professional image of the practitioner and that of the health professional establishment.

**Clothing:** work-wear should be freshly washed and ironed. Historically, this would be white for therapists, possibly with coloured trim. However, with changes in the market place there is a bounty of alternatives for you to choose from. A disposable plastic apron will protect your clothing from oil stains, a good idea especially if you are treating several babies one after the other.

**Footwear:** work does not lend itself well to 'high fashion' statements! Shoes should be fully enclosed with a low heel and clean – safety and comfort should be the priorities.

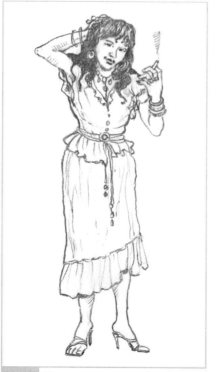 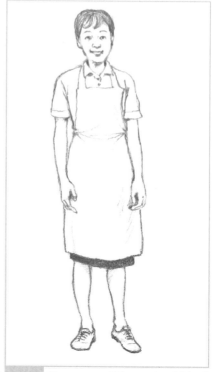

*How a practitioner should not look!*  *How a practitioner should look*

**Hair:** above all, hair should be kept clean. Long hair should be tied back; not only is it hygienic but it is practicable – let a baby grab a handful of your hair: it will surely be the last time you make that mistake!

**Jewellery:** should not be worn in the treatment room and in particular when massaging – rings, watches and bangles can scratch, and necklaces can be pulled. Jewellery is above all a perfect harbour for breeding bacteria and germs.

**Hands:** should be kept as soft as possible, by avoiding contact with chemicals, using hand creams, and protecting them as much as possible. Nails must be kept short and filed, as long or rough nails scratch a baby. Nail polish should not be worn because it attracts germs and bacteria. Hands must be washed with an anti-bacterial soap between each massage and the next.

**Personal hygiene:** is of paramount importance, particularly given the close proximity to clients that practitioners work in. Bathing or showering daily prevents embarrassing moments! Take care that your breath is as fresh as it should be, bearing in mind that food, drinks and smoking will affect it. Use breath fresheners during the day, clean your teeth after meals and avoid strong-smelling foods like garlic – certain smells tend to hang around longer than you expect!

Part of a health professional's job can be having to tell people that they have a 'personal hygiene' problem. There is nothing more difficult than having to say 'it can be very unpleasant to be close to you', and equally it is unpleasant to overhear such a comment. Try to avoid making such comments necessary!

## REFRESH YOUR KNOWLEDGE

1. What legislation is concerned with standards of hygiene in premises used for massage?

2. How does your appearance affect the 'professional image'?

3. What legislation promotes high standards of health and safety in the workplace?

4. Under the Health and Safety at Work Act, list three things the employer is responsible for, and three things the employee is responsible for.

5. Draw a picture of an appropriately dressed practitioner.

*for answers, see page 133.*

# Your practice notes

# Stages in Growth and Development of a Child

This part of the book is needed as underpinning knowledge for the qualification. That is to say that you don't need to 'know' this inside out and back to front, but you do need an awareness of the content. Having a good understanding of the growth and development of children will support your professionalism: just by looking, you will be able to closely identify the age of a child before being told, and be aware if a child is less or more advanced than they typically should be. It will mean you are more confident working with any baby/child.

## Reflex Actions

There are five core reflex actions, or spontaneous responses, that are checked for at birth. These are the suckling and swallowing, rooting, grasping, walking and startle, or 'Moro', reflexes. These reflexes are also used in the first few years of life as a measure of the child's development. As the child grows and develops, other influences in the body will help develop these reflexes and in most cases the child will learn to voluntary control them.

It is important that the practitioner is aware of these reflexes during massage; for example, sudden movements or loud noises will activate the startle reflex, the baby will throw his or her arms and legs out, possibly even arch the back, or when a finger is put into his or her hand it will be grasped.

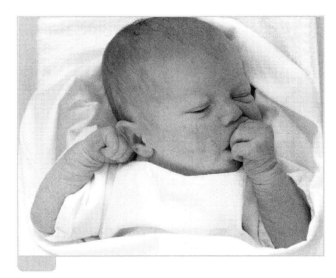

- **Suckling and swallowing** – when anything is put into a baby's mouth they will automatically suck and swallow.

- **Rooting** – babies turn towards their mother's nipple when gently touched on the cheek.

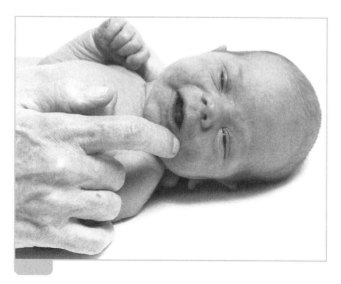

- **Grasping** – a baby's hand automatically grasps anything that is put into it.

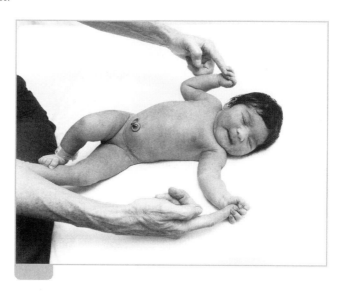

- **Walking** – held upright under the arms with feet touching a firm surface, babies make walking movements.

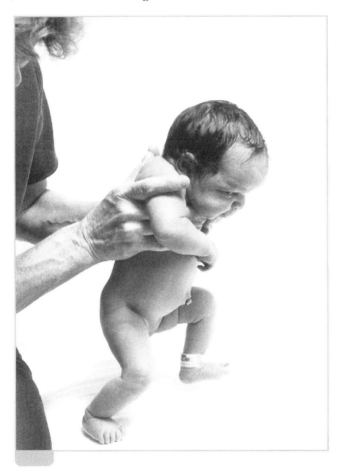

- **Startle** – a star shape is formed by babies when they are let go of suddenly.

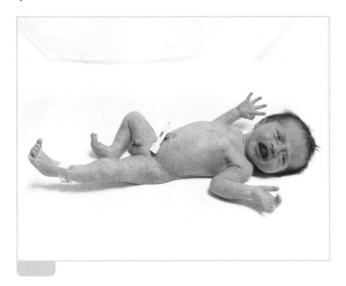

# Development 0–5 Years

These are the most formative years of a child's life: everything they see, hear and experience contributes along pre-programmed lines to the development of complex ideas, relationships, feelings and modes of expression.

## Newborn

From birth, a baby begins to use all of its senses to explore and learn about the new environment around them. A baby quickly recognises its mother or primary care-giver's smell and voice. Newborns focus on objects close to them and show a preference for human faces. They are alert to new sounds and smells, light and touch. All this information is sorted in the baby's remarkable data bank of new information until it needs to be re-called as the child grows and develops.

By one month babies are able follow you (and objects) around the room with their eyes, they can kick and wave their arms and will often imitate facial expressions. They often also start to smile in response to adult attention.

## Common features of this stage:

- kicking, stretching, moving the arms and legs and turning the head
- being aware of light and movement but is very short sighted
- crying when hungry or in pain.
- does not play
- usually clenches hands tight with thumbs in
- likes to be held close, cuddled and stroked.

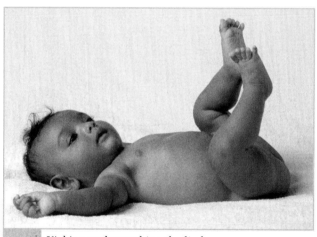

*Kicking and stretching the limbs*

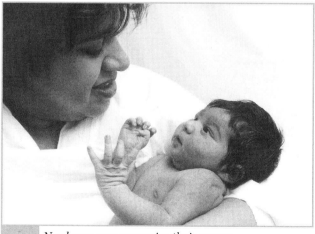

*Newborns can recognise their carers*

## Three Months

At about three months of age babies are beginning to show more interest in toys and objects. They are able to hold a rattle for a brief time before dropping it, and enjoy exploring different textures, for example a fluffy carpet. They also kick vigorously and clasp their hands together – demonstrating a combination of excited movements. They can recognise familiar situations and faces, and will gurgle with delight, often recognising their primary care-giver's face in photographs! Other vocal changes consist of various different cries, cooing and chuckling sounds. Emotionally, three-month-old babies show particular pleasure in loving attention, cuddles, being bathed and will stare at their carer during feeding.

## Common features of this stage:

- plays with fingers, grasping tightly
- smiles at people and toys with pleasure

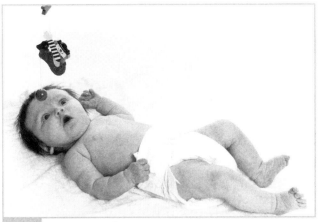
*Focuses on objects*

- gurgles and bubbles, holding 'conversation'
- lifts head in prone position
- responds to familiar situations.

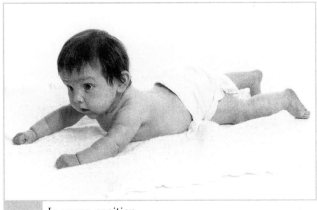
*In prone position*

## Six Months

As children become more aware of their surroundings, they extend their exploration by using their hands to touch, stroke and pat objects, often grabbing toys with both hands then transferring them to their mouths. They continue to find people, in particular, fascinating and begin to understand the meanings of such words as 'mama' or 'bye-bye'. They will often imitate sounds and will sometimes babble away to themselves in play. Socially, the six-month-old sometimes offers toys to others, becomes more wary of strangers and shows distress when their primary care-giver leaves the room. They also begin to recognise emotions, often laughing when another person does, or crying with another child.

### Common features of this stage:

- able to reach and grab items
- passes toys from one hand to the other
- makes a variety of sounds
- is able to focus fully as eyes work together now
- can sit up without being held
- begins exploring with rolling

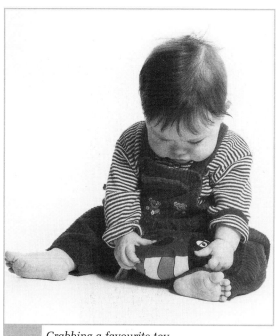
*Grabbing a favourite toy*

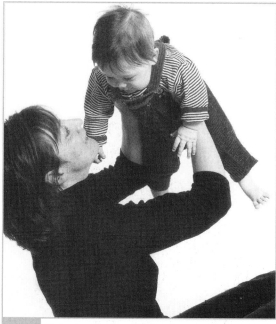
*Enjoying personal attention*

- laughs and chuckles with delight when they get attention.

## Nine Months

At nine months a child's exploring is vastly improved by his or her ability to shuffle on their bottom from one end of the room to the other, or crawl – often at incredible speeds! They will bounce in time to music, enjoying nursery rhymes and songs, as well as making noise by banging on boxes or other objects. Reaching forward they are able to grab and pick up an object, pulling it towards themselves and studying it closely. Although they prefer to be close to a familiar adult, nine-month-olds can play alone for periods of time. They are also beginning to show definite likes and dislikes, particularly for kinds of food.

## Common features of this stage:

- shuffles or crawls
- is often able to bounce to music
- is able to lean forward and pull objects close to them
- has a daily routine that can be understood
- imitates speech and gestures
- will play interactive games like 'peek-a-boo'.

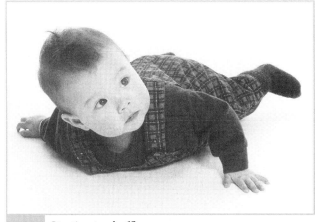

*Starting to shuffle*

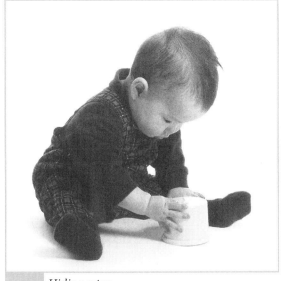

*Hiding a toy*

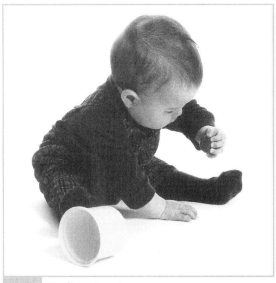

*Finding it again*

## One Year

As the child becomes more mobile their view of the world changes significantly. Clinging to the furniture for support they are often able to walk, as well as crawl, around rooms, thus increasing their exploration of their world further. Language, although still punctuated with unrecognisable words, begins to develop into conversation. They are able to understand, and respond to, simple instructions such as 'come here' or 'eat up'. By now there is often a favourite toy or object which is usually carried everywhere, but when forgotten or misplaced the child will sometimes become highly distressed. Children at this age can have fluctuating moods, and while often still shy of strangers, they can be warm and affectionate with familiar adults.

## Common features of this stage:

- crawls rapidly, often walks

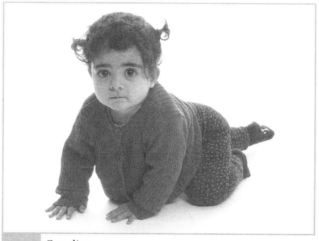

*Crawling*

- is usually shy with strangers
- recognises people and objects they know
- often has a favourite toy or blanket
- has a language that develops into conversation, although there are few recognisable words.

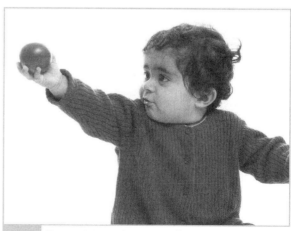

*Recognising a favourite object*

## Eighteen Months

A good sense of balance enables children at this age to walk well, run, and climb up and down stairs unaided. Their fine motor co-ordination has developed enough to enable them to pick up small objects, such as crayons or pens. They also often begin to show a preference for one hand (see below). Developing their own characteristics and personality, they are able to understand simple commands and through this often show their desire for independence! They will also often refer to themselves by name, e.g. 'Zoë wants to play'. In play, eighteen-month-olds enjoy sand and water play, matching and sorting games, singing and action rhymes and painting.

## Common features of this stage:

- walks well
- is able to climb and descend stairs with help
- obeys simple commands
- feeds themself
- is often ready for potty training
- begins to show preference for one or other hand.

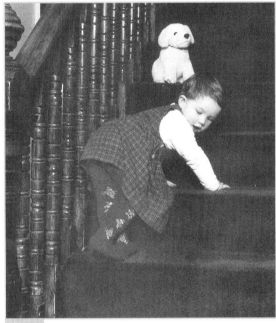

*Climbing unaided downstairs*

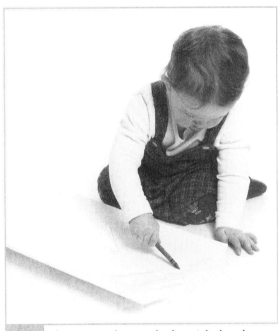

*Showing preference for her right hand*

## Two Years

The phrase 'time of self-expression' springs to mind! Two-year-olds will demonstrate strong emotions – bursting into tears, laughing or crying in sympathy – as they begin to express how they feel. They are frustrated easily when they can't achieve something, are prevented from doing something or are having difficulty in expressing themselves. However, children of this age also find great pleasure in naming objects and actions such as 'step', 'doll' or 'wave' and it is also the age when imagination and creativity really begins to show. They want to be as independent as possible, try to please you with their expressions and words, exploring their environment, running and jumping, laughing and kicking in an exhausting and curious way.

## Common features of this stage:

- can run, climb, dance, kick and throw a ball
- uses words and actions to clearly express themself

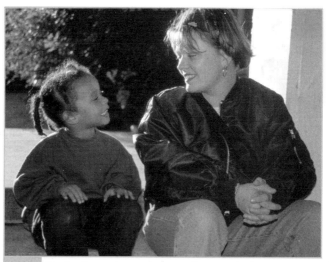
*Beginning to have conversations*

- can make simple sentences of two or three words
- can see as far as an adult
- demonstrates strong emotions, often referred to as 'temper tantrums'.

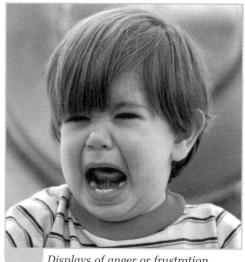
*Displays of anger or frustration*

## Two and a Half Years

At two and a half children seem to have little or no sense of danger as they will often charge around all day – walking, running and climbing. They often may not sleep through the night and are constantly asking questions 'why, who, what?' with one answer leading to the next question . . . and so it goes on! Picture books become more fascinating than ever, often they will read their own story, even if the book is upside down, and will talk audibly and intelligibly to themselves when playing. I was reading the Sunday paper when my two-and-a-half-year-old picked up the colour supplement and studied it hard waiting for me to notice, then smiled, fluttered her eyelashes and continued to read!

### Common features of this stage:

- very active, has little sense of danger
- asks questions
- enjoys picture books and being read to
- can jump with two feet together from a low step.

## Three Years

At three years of age children really begin to interact *with* other children, they start to play with other children rather than along side them, and making their first friends. Using their imaginations they can tell stories, illustrate recognisable shapes and experiment with colour and will use any excuse to use a pair of scissors! Socially, three-year-olds tend to enjoy doing things unaided, helping adults with chores like tiding up or sweeping, and they can think about things from other people's viewpoint.

### Common features of this stage:

- plays with other children, understands sharing
- can jump and stand on one foot
- tells stories with imagination
- uses scissors.

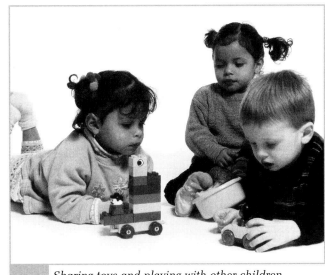
*Sharing toys and playing with other children*

### Four Years

Most four-year-olds have developed their physical skills to enable them to walk down stairs as an adult would, bend from the waist to pick up objects, enjoy climbing on trees and frames and maintain good balance. In play, dressing up and role playing goes a long way towards feeding their now inquisitive imaginations, often re-enacting stories from books and television and making up their own stories and characters. A four-year-old's use of language includes asking numerous questions about how things work and what happens if, etc., as well as being able to recite nursery rhymes, tell long stories and state their full name and address mostly without mistakes.

### Common features of this stage:

- independent and capable
- walks with a swinging step, and can hop and jump
- uses speech which is easy to understand.

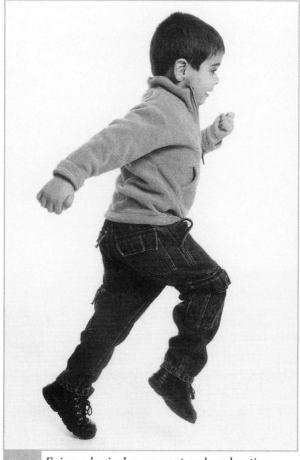

*Enjoys physical movement and exploration*

## Five Years

Children at this stage of development show independence in everyday skills such as dressing, cleaning their teeth and using the toilet. They are learning self-control, for example how to wait and how to take turns, and thus developing a more sophisticated understanding of social interaction. Five-year-olds understand the social rules of their culture, and instinctively help other children when they are distressed. They also enjoy being able to please, to show, to tell and to share by showing what they can do, have done and what they want to do. Physically, five-year-olds tend to show good balance, have increased agility, show good co-ordination and use a variety of play equipment such as swings and slides.

## Common features of this stage:

- learns self-control, the need to wait, how to share and how to take it in turns
- is very independent
- skips, plays ball games confidently
- can draw recognisable houses, people, trees etc.

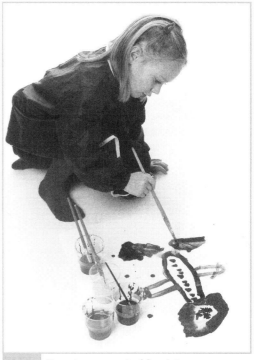

*Drawing recognisable pictures*

## REFRESH YOUR KNOWLEDGE

1. What are the five reflexes babies are born with?

2. Name two things you would expect a six-month-old baby to be able to do.

3. Why is it important as a practitioner to be able to recognise a child's developmental age?

*for answers, see page 133–4*

# Your practice notes

# How Babies Communicate

Communication is an essential part of most people's daily lives. It helps people express their needs, to build and maintain relationships and to interact. It is a skill that is often taken for granted but one that plays a vital role in a baby or child's development. Often the term communication is misinterpreted to refer only to 'formal' communication such as written and spoken language, however is used in a variety of ways, such as body language and facial expression.

A baby's communication skills begin long before its birth. Pregnant women often speak of their developing foetuses moving in the uterus giving them a nudge in the side or under the ribs to let them know it does not like the position they are in. It has also been reported that unborn babies can hear sound frequencies from the external environment, for example a baby will sometimes move its body in response to its mother's speech or in time to musical beats.

## CASE STUDY

*Antoinette's five-year-old son, Chris, started singing along to a piece of music that she had not played since she had given birth to him. He could not remember ever having heard it before, and yet he quite clearly knew the piece enough to hum the tune and recognise the chorus. People all over the world have, and continue to, report the same phenomena.*

Although children begin to understand and respond to language and vocal sounds from birth, the art of speech follows much later. Semi-understandable or recognisable speech begins to develop at about twelve months, developing from single words to stringing whole sentences together – the beginnings of conversation (see pages 20–9).

## CASE STUDY *cont.*

*Antoinette: "Chris and his sister Ruby followed the same learning pattern with their speech. They mastered the idea of stringing words together at about twelve months, grasping the concept of sentences, however they promptly became completely nonsensical – we couldn't understand a word they were saying! This lasted for about six months or so before it all suddenly came together and we could all understand each other again!"*

Prior to mastering the art of speech, communication with a child or baby takes its form in a different way: through body language, touch, facial expressions, holding, rocking, singing and listening. It is thought that around 60 per cent of communication is expressed through non-verbal communication whereby we interpret and respond to others' gestures, facial expressions and body movements. Learning to interpret and respond to babies and young children's non-verbal communication is an important aspect of being a successful and confident massage practitioner.

reflect

Think about the expression 'its not what you say, its how you say it'. Does the **way** we say things have an effect on the outcome? Think about the way we communicate with babies and young children, is it different from the way we talk to each other? During a massage routine, do you think the way we communicate will have an impact on the massage?

For some people communicating with a child or baby is a natural instinct, but not for everyone. Many adults feel that communicating with babies is the hardest thing in the world, saying that babies always cry when they hold them or try to play with them. To overcome this we need to do two things: firstly gain an understanding of what babies are trying to communicate and the methods they use, and secondly gain confidence so that we are ready for interaction.

## Understanding baby communication
### Infant activity levels
Babies and children will use different form of communicate depending on their current mood or level of activity. The different types of infant activity levels can be defined into six categories:

- **Deep sleep** – there is little or no movement, breathing is regulated, the eyes remain still
- **Light sleep** – some body movement will be noticeable with rapid eye movement, smiles or whimpers which are often associated with dreaming
- **Drowsy state** – the eyes, when open, will appear glazed and heavy, usually as a child is waking, or as he or she is about to fall asleep. The level of activity will increase upon awakening and decrease upon sleep, breathing will be irregular and responses delayed
- **Alert state** – a baby will be at its most attentive state here, focusing hard on people and objects, using many facial expressions, for example its face lights up when it focuses on its carer. This is the ideal time for massage as the baby is alert, well rested and happy

- **Active alert state** – the baby is busy with lots of movement, sensitive to stimuli, but can be 'fussy' at times.

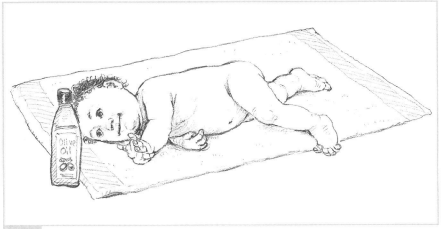

*The active alert state is not always the easiest time to get baby to stay in one place for a massage, but the best time for fun and games!*

During massage – which is usually recommended while the baby is in an alert state or an active alert state – it is important to respond to the baby in the right way. Knowing what the baby wants is half the battle, this is why interpreting the child's non-verbal communication becomes so important.

Think about body posture and movements. When you are with a friend and they want to be alone, what do they do? Babies do the same, they turn away from you, the only difference is that they do not use verbal communication to reinforce their actions. They are more subtle, therefore observation needs to be much more focused and will need to consider all the types of non-verbal communication available: body posture, movement, eye contact and facial expressions.

## Identifying Crying

Before babies and young children learn to laugh and giggle, their only form of verbal communication is crying. Although it can take a while and it can be challenging, identifying different types of cries enables the practitioner to master the needs of a baby. There are very distinct differences between a hungry baby crying for food and one that crying in pain, anger or from tiredness.

- **Hunger:** Typically this is an urgent, short cry that, if left unattended, can turn into frustration and anger. It is not usually accompanied with tears, but is loud and shrill, often the baby will shake as he or she becomes more upset.
- **Pain:** A sharp, piercing and intense cry demanding immediate response – once heard, never forgotten!

- **Anger:** A sustained low-pitched cry often accompanied by a red face, tight lips and clenched fists.
- **Tiredness**: This is often a whimpering, non-urgent and non-rhythmical cry, accompanied by the baby rubbing its eyes, feeling for its ears, or sucking its fingers.

**SAFE PRACTICE**

*If a baby starts to whimper or cry during a massage then the treatment should be stopped.*

**CASE STUDY**

*Desh, a massage practitioner, took his six-week-old daughter, Sam, to his son's school to give the children a demonstration of baby massage. Although there were thirty or so children surrounding Sam, she was so tired that she fell asleep during the massage. Instead of her usual whimper she lay there quietly looking at the children. Desh soon realised that Sam had drifted off to sleep, so he stopped the massage and tucked her up quietly in a blanket for an hour – the children were fascinated! This is a good example of how a baby was so relaxed by the massage that she didn't let her carer know how tired she was.*

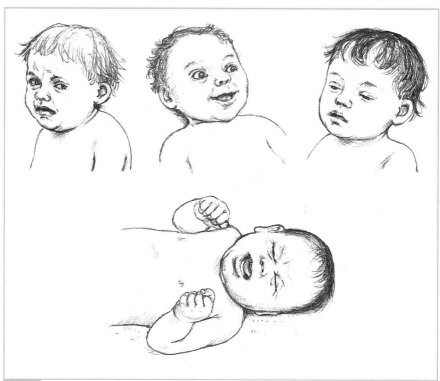

*Can you tell from their facial expressions, and body posture what these children are trying to communicate?*

# Ready for interaction

The following table outlines some of the most common forms of communication children and babies use to let you know that they are ready for interaction, or not:

| COMMUNICATION | READY FOR INTERACTION | NOT READY FOR INTERACTION |
| --- | --- | --- |
| Facial expressions | Smiling, eyes widen & 'sparkle' | Eyes turn away, not smiling, possibly grimacing or frowning |
| Head & eye movements | Turning towards you, continuous eye contact | Turning away, possibly closing eyes, yawning |
| Body movements | Excited movements, relaxed limbs | Arching back, raising shoulders, increased movement which can be jerky or erratic. Pulling away, trying to turn away |
| Hands | Hands are sometimes open, but fingers are relaxed | Clenched fists |
| Verbal | Bubbly, cooing sounds, giggles and laughs | Whimpering or crying |

There are no 'magic' tricks that are needed to work and communicate with babies and young children. The practitioner however will need to be a good listener, be attentive to the child's needs and create environments and situations that help the child to feel at ease. Communication is a two-way process, the practitioner will also communicate his or her feelings to the child through body language and facial expressions. Feeling confident, calm and ready for massage will help the child or baby to feel the same (see pages 66–9 for exercises to help the practitioner feel ready for interaction). If you can learn to read the signs a baby is giving you this will not only support your professionalism, but will also improve your confidence in working with babies and children, which in turn will make you a much better practitioner, and also inspire confidence in the carer or parent.

# Your practice notes

# Related Anatomy and Physiology

It is important to have a clear understanding of anatomy and physiology in order to ensure safe practice. The simple action of massage movements performed on the body of a baby will affect the physiological response from that body. It is necessary to understand the effects of the massage movements because it explains why it is so important to follow the guidance of the massage routine. Without this knowledge you might perform massage movements against the blood flow or against the digestive system with damaging effect.

## The Growth of the Skeleton

At birth the skeleton consists mainly of **cartilage**, a soft bendy substance. As growth proceeds the cartilage gradually develops into bone, leaving only a small amount in joints, ears, the nose and throat. This process is known as **ossification** and is completed by a child's late teens. Up to this point children's bones remain relatively soft and are therefore susceptible to fractures, the bone bending rather than breaking.

Ossification proceeds in regular stages making it possible to estimate fairly accurately the age of a child from a skeleton.

### The Effects of Massage on the Growth of the Skeleton

Joint mobility, flexibility and strength are increased when massage is performed regularly. Pressure against the **periosteum**, which surrounds the bones, stimulates the blood circulation to them. This feeds and nourishes the bones and joints in the neighbouring area.

reflect

Remember the babies' bones are very soft! Ask the carer or parent to hold his or her finger out in front of the baby and run the pad of the thumb gently over the surface of the back of the baby's hand. Can they feel the metacarpals?

# The Blood

The number of red blood cells required prior to birth is far less than that after birth, therefore the additional cells are broken down and the **haemoglobin** is stored in the liver. **Vitamin K** is needed by the liver for the production of **prothrombin**, one of the elements necessary for clotting blood. To assist the baby's low clotting power, vitamin K is administered at birth to most babies.

## *The Effects of Massage on the Blood*

All massage movements affect the circulation of the blood, even superficial effleurage, which produces a contraction of the **capillary walls** in the skin, having a soothing and cooling effect on the body. Arteries are too deep-seated to be truly affected, however the **venous circulation** is increased bringing fresh nutrients and oxygen to the cells as well as removing waste products, such as carbon dioxide. It is essential to apply movements with any pressure in a **centripetal direction**, that is, towards the heart, where the venous trunks return deoxygenated blood to the right side of the heart.

reflect

Blood flows around our bodies reaching every extremity and filling the tissues with oxygen and nutrients. As you massage the flow will increase and the colour of the skin will 'pink up' in response, this is the blood filling those tiny spaces with goodness.

# The Muscular System

Voluntary and involuntary muscles alike continue to strengthen and develop throughout adolescence needing nourishment from the blood and exercise to develop fully. Involuntary muscles work on their own: the heart, gut and bladder. In massage we are mainly concerned with voluntary muscles, also called **striated (striped) muscles** because of their arrangement of muscle fibres. They produce their effect by shortening in length (contraction). These muscles are distributed throughout the body, attached by tendons to bones, and so enabling conscious movement, like walking, running and jumping.

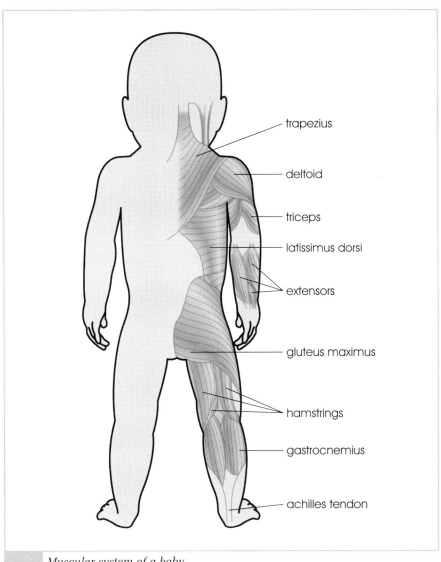

- trapezius
- deltoid
- triceps
- latissimus dorsi
- extensors
- gluteus maximus
- hamstrings
- gastrocnemius
- achilles tendon

*Muscular system of a baby*

## The Effects of Massage on the Muscular System

Massage is particularly effective after physical exercise, for example after a baby's bath, and before bedtime. This is because massage increases the circulation in a muscle, relieving accumulated products such as lactic acid, a waste product of muscle activity. If **lactic acid** is allowed to accumulate it can lead to muscle fatigue or cramp. The increased blood supply brings about an increase in heat, resulting in the whole body feeling warmer and more relaxed. Because a baby's muscles are developing continually at a rapid pace, massaging babies increases the development of their muscles, enabling them to grow and function at the optimum level.

# Foetal Circulation/Respiration

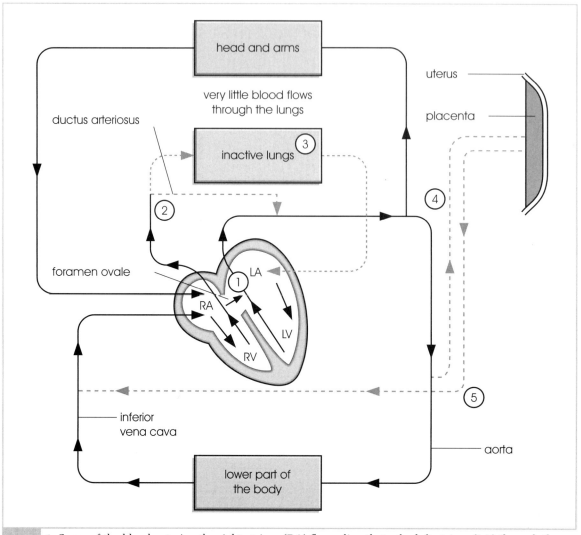

1 *Some of the blood entering the right atrium (RA) flows directly to the left atrium (LA) through the* **foramen ovale**.

2 *Most of the blood from the right ventricle (RV) flows through the* **ductus arteriosus**.

3 *Very little blood flows through the lungs.*

4 *The umbilical* **artery** *branches from the aorta.*

5 *Blood in the umbilical vein goes to the inferior vena cava.*

The first function to be established at birth is breathing. This involves a re-routing of the blood and expansion of the lungs. The lungs of a baby in the **uterus** are collapsed until birth. The **alveoli cells** secrete a substance called **surfactant** which prevents the walls of the alveoli from adhering. Once the first breath is drawn the lungs expand and fill with oxygen.

The process begins with the separation of the **placenta** from the uterine wall. The umbilical artery then contracts and stops blood from flowing to the placenta. The blood continues to flow through the umbilical vein until most of the baby's blood has returned from the placenta to the baby. Once the pulsating movements cease, the cord is clamped and cut. Blood then circulates through the lungs.

The fall in oxygen and rise in carbon dioxide stimulates the baby to gasp air, so that the lungs expand and breathing begins. The **foramen ovale** and **ductus arteriosus** close. The process is complete and the baby breathes independently from the mother. The umbilical cord dries and sloughs off between six and ten days later. During this time it is kept clean and dry to avoid infection. Sterile powder is no longer used as it is thought to be **carcinogenic** (cancer forming).

## The Effects of Massage on the Lungs

The condition, strength and function of the lungs can be improved through the mobilisation of the joints of the **thorax**. Gaseous interchange is increased, ridding the body of carbon dioxide and replenishing the lungs with fresh oxygen. We have already learnt that a baby's circulation is increased, and this includes that of the lungs. Therefore there is an increase in nutrition maintaining the elasticity of the alveoli, and enabling expiration of any mucus or foreign bodies.

reflect

Listen to baby breathing with the carer or parent. In excitement its breaths will increase, as relaxation takes over its breaths will slow; how long did this take to happen for the baby? As you and the carer peform more massages they will notice the difference from treatment to treatment.

# The Lymphatic System

Newborn babies inherit their mother's immunity, which remains passive for some weeks before they are able to produce an active immunity. Before birth, **lymphocytes** migrate to the **thymus gland**, mature and develop into activated **T-lymphocytes**, able to respond to antigens encountered elsewhere in the body. The node is situated behind the **sternum** close to the heart in the **thoracic cavity**, extending upwards into the root of the neck. Although large in infants it does not grow as rapidly as the body and therefore remains proportionate to the need of the immune system. After puberty the node decreases and its exact function in the adult is uncertain.

## *The Effects of Massage on the Lymphatic System*

Experiments have shown that massage increases the **lymphatic flow**; petrissage movements serve to squeeze the lymphatic spaces and effleurage moves it to the nearest gland. Fresh lymph seeps through the walls of capillary blood vessels to feed the tissues and absorb waste products. Movement of lymph is dependent upon external forces, gravity, muscle contraction or massage. If there is a local infection, the lymph fluid will help to pass it on to the lymph glands, therefore massage is contra-indicated for local infections.

**SAFE PRACTICE**

*Remember to direct your movements towards the lymphatic nodes.*

# The Nervous System

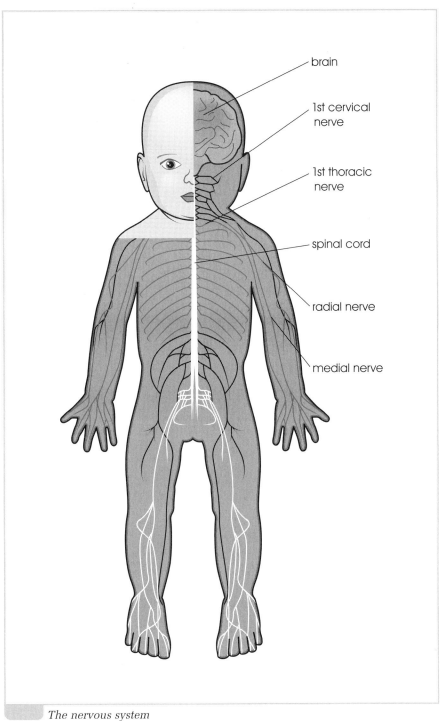

brain

1st cervical nerve

1st thoracic nerve

spinal cord

radial nerve

medial nerve

*The nervous system*

The centre of the nervous system is the spine and brain, receiving and sending messages all over the body through a complex system of interconnected nerve cells called **neurones**.

Neurones are divided into three types: **sensory neurones**, which convey information from the body's sense organs; **integrative neurones**, which process information received; and **motor neurones**, that initiate voluntary and involuntary actions. The nervous system is essential to sensory perception, pain and pleasure, control of movement, and the regulation of body functions like breathing.

## The Effects of Massage on the Nervous System

Effleurage and petrissage tend to have a sedative and soothing effect, causing the nerves to respond reflexively to the gentle stimulation and thus induce relaxation.

There is a local effect on the sensory nerves, which convey messages (such as temperature changes and pain) from the sense organs to the central nervous system; as well as a local effect on the motor nerves, which convey messages from the central nervous system and supply muscles to bring about movement. Experiments show that massage can affect the autonomic nervous system, the involuntary part of the nervous system (controlling the functions carried out automatically).

reflect

Hopefully the carer will notice, the first time he/she massages, the reaction of the baby, who will automatically feel a sense of calm take over and will slip into the massage as if it were the most natural thing in the world! The carer may even find him or herself 'slipping away' with them, the power of the massage on the sensory neurones bringing 'goose bumps' to their skin, too!

# The Skin

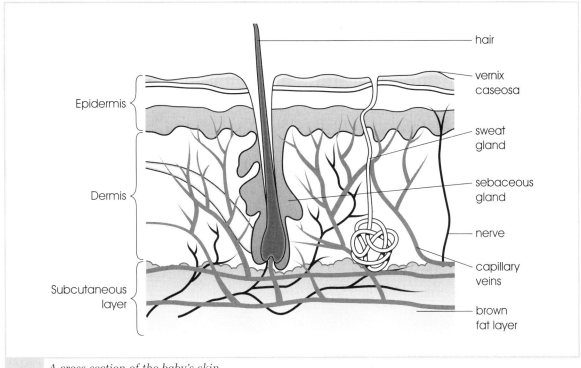

Epidermis

Dermis

Subcutaneous layer

hair

vernix caseosa

sweat gland

sebaceous gland

nerve

capillary veins

brown fat layer

*A cross-section of the baby's skin*

A baby's skin is fine and delicate; pre-term babies are usually soft and wrinkly, whereas post-term babies tend to be dry and flaky. The skin is easily irritated, abraded and infected. Babies are born with a substance called **vernix caseosa** covering them, secreted by the sebaceous glands. This acts as a lubricant during birth, protecting the skin and helping a baby to retain heat.

**Lanugo,** a downy fluff of very fine hair is also present at birth and usually more obvious on pre-term babies than full-term. Full-term babies are born with an insulating layer of **brown fat**, which acts as fuel to supply extra heat when required.

## The Effects of Massage on the Skin

Massage aids and increases skin shedding (**desquamation**), avoiding a build-up of dead skin cells, thus improving the overall condition of the skin and its ability to absorb nutrients. **Sweat** and **sebaceous glands** are stimulated, increasing the output of sweat and **sebum**, helping to keep the skin soft and supple, improving texture and its resistance to infection.

reflect

Ask the carer to tell you how the skin feels and if there are any changes from performing the massage

# The Digestive System

All the nutrients, essential amino acids, vitamins and elements required for survival whilst in the womb are fed pre-digested to a baby though the umbilical cord. Once born, babies have to learn to digest before their stomach's contents can be absorbed and utilised.

Babies are born with an immature **enzyme system**, used to break down fat, starch and sugars, which means an overload results in diarrhoea. Maturation of the enzymes occurs within a baby's first few days, having not been required in the uterus for digestion.

There is considerable evidence to suggest that many components of human breast milk are more readily absorbed than the equivalent components in formula milk.

## Elimination

Shortly after birth, and sometimes during birth, babies pass their first stool, **meconium**, which is present in the intestine from about the sixteenth week of intra-uterine life. It is dark green to black in colour and composed of **bile** pigment, fatty acids and **epithelial cells**. From then on babies have normal bowel movements, unless the digestive system is overloaded.

## Colostrum

A mother's breast secretes colostrum for the first two or three days after birth, which increases progressively in volume and alters in composition, until by the third or fourth day milk is being produced together with colostrum. Colostrum is a translucent fluid, high in protein and lower in fat and sugar than milk. The large **globulin** proportion includes **immunoglobulins**, some of which may be absorbed by the infant. **IGA** is the most important of the globulins, acting as a protection in the bowel against viruses and bacteria.

## The Function of the Liver

The liver plays a major role in the elimination of toxic products, as well as working as a biochemical factory in which new substances and proteins necessary for tissue growth are prepared. **Bilirubin** is a breakdown product of haemoglobin, normally present by the fourth day (although in pre-term babies by the sixth or seventh day).

## The Urinary System

Excretion from the foetus takes place through the umbilical cord until birth. The bladder is usually emptied at birth and can take up to 24 hours to re-fill and empty again. The kidneys are inefficient at excreting fluids and do not function effectively until the level of fluid consumption increases sufficiently.

## The Effects of Massage on the Digestive System

Massage is effective in stimulating the **colon**, and so aiding digestion, although the movements are actually applied to the overlying muscles of the abdominal wall. Massage of the colon should always follow a clockwise direction, the natural flow of the contents of the colon. The movement of the involuntary muscle of the colon is called **peristalsis**. Peristaltic movement is increased by pressure extended on the stomach wall, and on the small and large intestine. Kneading of the **alimentary tract** is particularly effective in stimulating peristaltic action.

Massaging of the liver stimulates cell activity. Slow deep manipulations produce more bile, which is stored in the **gall bladder** until required. A baby's metabolism is increased, and as a result more waste products and heat are produced. Both **colic** and constipation are gently relieved by abdominal massage. Experiments have shown that there is an increase in the output of urine, containing nitrogen, inorganic phosphorus and chloride, particularly after abdominal massage.

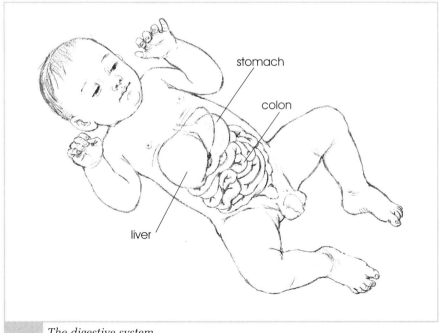

*The digestive system*

1. Why are a baby's lungs collapsed in the uterus?

2. Name the two ducts which close when breathing begins at birth.

3. Why is the clotting power of a baby's blood low at birth?

4. Name two functions of brown fat.

*for answers, see page 134*

*Note:* See page 132 for Baby anatomy and physiology assessment.

# Your practice notes

# Contra-indications to Baby Massage

A contra-indication is something that prevents you from performing a massage. In some cases this could be a temporary condition, like not waking a sleeping baby, and in others it could be more serious. It could be that by gaining permission from a baby's doctor, the massage can be carried out at a later date.

Whatever the situation, it is important to check carefully for contra-indications before proceeding with massage treatment.

Listed below are the contra-indications associated with baby massage. Ensure that carers are aware of these so theat they can practise safe massage on their own.

## SAFE PRACTICE

*If you are not sure, don't do it.*

A contra-indication exists where a baby:

- has skin disorders or infections. It is important not to make the condition any worse or to spread it

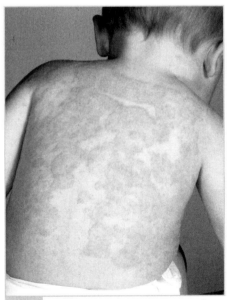

*Atropic eczema is a contra-indication to massage*

- gets upset. If your baby gets upset during massage, stop and try again another time. Some babies take a little time to get used to it. **Do not massage forcibly or against a baby's will**
- has been recently immunised. After immunisation, wait 48 hours to see how it affects the child. If there are no problems, massage but avoid the injection site until it is no longer sensitive
- is asleep. Never wake a baby for massage. A sleeping baby should be left alone or they will get irritable and associate massage with this
- is hungry. If a baby is hungry, feed them first, then massage later, waiting at least half an hour to allow for digestion, otherwise the baby will vomit the feed
- has had recent surgery – avoid the area affected, and to be safe always check with a baby's doctor first
- is currently undergoing medical treatment (unless doctor's permission is given first)
- has a dysfunction of the nervous system
- has had a recent haemorrhage
- has swellings or cuts
- has had recent fractures and sprains.

If contra-indications are established, a physician's approval must be obtained by the parent or guardian prior to any massage being given.

**SAFE PRACTICE**

*It is important that all contra-indications are fully explained to the parent or carer and that a disclaimer is signed by them.*

# Massaging Children With Special Needs

The term 'special needs' (also referred to as particular or individual needs) is used in a variety of ways across different settings. It is often used to describe people with an impairment or medical condition who have particular needs and requirements. In this chapter we are going to look briefly at some of the impairments and medical conditions that we may come across during our work as a massage practitioners, how we can work with children and their parents or carers who have individual needs, and where possible how we can use massage as a support. This is not a definitive chapter on special needs; it is an introduction aimed at providing enough knowledge to give you the confidence to talk to and work with parents or carers and their children with special needs. (Please see page 140 for names of organisations that can offer more information and advice.)

**SAFE PRACTICE**

*Always get the support of the child's GP prior to starting any massage treatment to ensure that the child has no contra-indications to massage.*

## Sensory Impairments

Sensory impairment refers to the loss of one or more of our five senses: sights, smell, hearing, touch or taste. Often if one or more of these senses are lost then the remaining senses become more acute or developed. For example, if sight is lost then the sense of touch can be developed to read Braille and the acuteness of hearing will support the child who is unable to see a car coming, hearing the car coming instead.

reflect

Spend a few moments working in pairs. One of you close your eyes while the other gently massages. Discuss your experiences; did you jump when you were first touched? Consider how you might adjust your massage technique to improve the experience.

## Visual impairment

Visual impairment can vary from complete to partial blindness, affecting a child from birth, or as the result of an infection, such as measles, later in life. Massage can be particularly beneficial to a visually impaired child, helping them to feel secure in their environment and increase the bonding between carer and child.

It is important to explain each step of the process carefully to the child, using the voice to indicate your intention to change from talking to massage. Taking the child's hand and placing it on the part of the body to be massaged also prevents the child from getting a fright and becoming anxious. Describing the different body parts to the child helps him or her to understand what massage is, as does allowing the child to feel the oils or lotions that will be used. It can also work well to ask the child to massage your leg or arm, once you have explained how to, before beginning the routines.

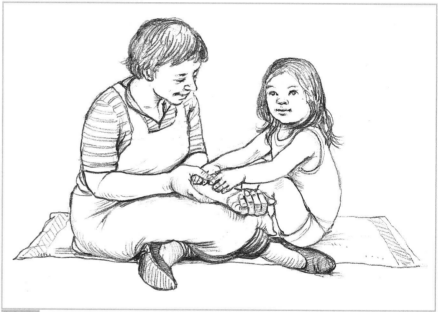

*Let the child massage your own arm before you begin the routine*

## Hearing impairments

As with visual impairments, hearing impairments can vary from slight to profound, and may result from injuries or infections before, during or after birth. Demonstrating massage to the baby or child, using yourself, the carer or a doll, is a good way of explaining to the child what massage is. Some children may be able to communicate using sign language. When demonstrating make sure that eye contact is kept with the child by yourself or the carer. Use facial expressions to support your movements – keep it light and happy and the child will relax with you.

## Loss of a limb

Losing a limb is often the result of an injury or accident, but can also be the result of an infection or disease necessitating amputation. Before beginning the massage always consult the child's parent or carer before removing any prostheses to ensure that it is removed and stored correctly during the massage. During massage don't 'ignore' the affected limb – treat the child in same way you would any other. For example, when massaging a child whose right hand has been amputated, follow the arm massage routine (pages 90–1) until you reach the point of amputation, gently massage the area, improvising if necessary. Follow this with a full hand and arm massage to the child's left arm and hand. Massaging the amputated area has particular physiological benefits as it encourages the supply of fresh blood and lymph to the area keeping it healthy, whilst simultaneously stimulating the nerves. Psychologically the massage can enhance the child's sense of security and acceptance.

# Down's Syndrome

Down's syndrome is a genetic condition (meaning present from birth) caused by the presence of extra genetic material. Down's syndrome does not affect all children in the same way, but many will have similar characteristics including: hearing loss, visual impairments or heart problems, and can be prone to respiratory and other infections. They often also have poor muscle tone and tend to have shorter hands and feet.

**SAFE PRACTICE**

*Approximately 50 per cent of children with Down's syndrome have heart defects, therefore its important to get their GPs approval before proceeding with the massage.*

**CASE STUDY**

*Neil worked with Down's syndrome children at his first teaching college: "they were wonderful, loving, affectionate and caring. Although we only did hand and arm massage they loved it, telling me it made their skin feel nice! I remember distinctly that they all had incredibly dry skin, the use of a good olive oil on a weekly basis made a huge difference and the condition of their nails improved immensely!"*

## Spina Bifida

Spina bifida is a congenital disorder in which the lower vertebrae of the spine do not develop fully, leaving part of the spinal cord exposed. In severe cases the child suffers a loss of sensation or the use of his or her lower limbs. Many children remain incontinent, some children may rely on mobility aids and some may require support to stand or sit.

The treatment of gentle massage can promote a feeling of well being, stimulate the circulation and help support the digestive system. Any existing sensation to the lower half of the body will be enhanced by the massage giving pleasure and awareness to the area.

## Childhood Cancer

One in every 600 children under the age of fifteen develops cancer. Although there is much speculation surrounding radiation, chemicals, infection and electro-magnetic fields there is no consensus as to the causes of childhood cancer. Allopathic (conventional) treatment is often invasive, with painful side effects and can take place over long periods of time, effecting the whole family.

As massage increases movement through the body's circulatory and lymphatic systems, massage can be beneficial physiologically. It can also have psychological benefits by providing an opportunity for deeper bonding between carer and child, as well as promoting well-being during this traumatic illness.

## Cystic Fibrosis

Cystic fibrosis is an inherited disease whereby a defective gene causes the body to produce an abnormally thick, sticky mucus that clogs the lungs and leads to life-threatening lung infections. These thick secretions also obstruct the pancreas, preventing digestive enzymes from reaching the intestines to help break down and absorb food. Children with this illness suffer reoccurring chest infections, sinus and breathing difficulties. Early diagnosis and careful management of treatment can sustain life into early adulthood. Providing GP approval has been given the potential benefits of massage to these children is enormous. Carefully applied thumb stroking (see page 92) across the chest will effectively drain the alveoli sacs in the lungs giving relief to the child by in aiding the drainage of the mucus from the lungs.

# Your practice notes

# PART TWO:
# The practice of massage

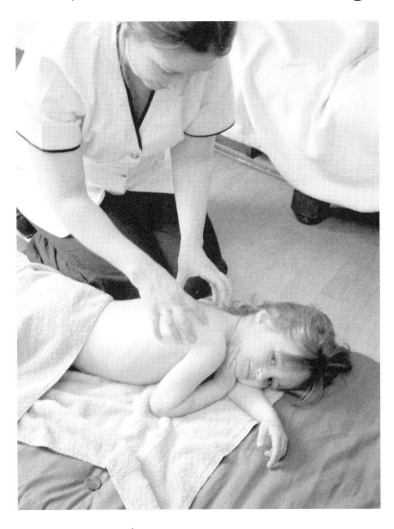

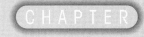
# Preparing for Massage

## Hygienic Baby Massage Treatment

Hygiene is not so much a set of rules, as an attitude of mind. Competence in terms of hygiene will prevent cross-infection between masseur and baby. It is of the utmost importance that, when treating or demonstrating massage on several babies in a group, hygiene practice is followed, because cross-infection can easily take place between babies, as their immunity is not well established.

The code of practice for hygiene in beauty salons and clinics, published by the VTCT, is the major industry code dealing with hygiene in all its aspects. Local authorities may also impose a licensing regime through by-laws.

### Guidelines

- The massage area should be kept clean, neat and well ventilated.
- Changing mats should be kept sanitised, and in preference a baby's own changing mat should be used.
- Ensure the floor is clean and dry.
- Fresh, clean towels should be used for each baby.
- Babies should be clean before undergoing massage.
- Cuts and abrasions should be covered (whether the practitioner's own or a baby's).
- Hands should be washed before and after massage.
- A surgical mask should be worn if you are suffering from a cold, to prevent transferring germs.
- Jewellery should not be worn.
- Any rubbish should be placed in a plastic lined bin.

These rules of hygiene vary depending on the situation, i.e. teaching a group, an individual, or with your own baby.

**SAFE PRACTICE**

*Remember, with groups there is a much higher risk of cross-infection.*

## Massage Support

There are a couple of ways to massage babies to ensure that they are both comfortable and safe. Do not massage on a high plinth or anywhere that babies could fall from. The following are best:

- the floor, on a clean, dry towel. Place a baby-changing mat underneath for extra comfort and to protect the floor should the baby urinate
- either on your or the carer's lap with legs outstretched, or lying across the lap and held in the arms. Small babies feel more secure if in contact with the parent
- on a bed. It is possible to massage babies on a towel on a bed, but place them in the centre and across the bed. It is not advisable for babies to be 'mobile' as they could easily fall. Note: beauty therapy 'beds' are not suitable to use.

**SAFE PRACTICE**

*Never leave a baby unattended! The floor or a lap is recommended for optimum safety.*

## Preparation for Massage

It is important to 'set the scene' for massage, as well as ensure that all safety checks are completed prior to it. The room must be warm and have adequate ventilation; germs flourish in a stuffy hot room. The light must not be too bright; babies hate really bright lights and it doesn't support a relaxing atmosphere for massage. Before commencing massage ensure that you and the carer have washed your hands thoroughly with an anti-bacterial soap and that hands are warm to touch.

You need to be undisturbed for at least half an hour, so: if there is a phone in the room turn off the ringer or unplug it; make sure nothing is left in the oven that needs 'turning' in ten minutes; or that a friend/colleague isn't due to call round at some time in the next twenty minutes. Not only will this spoil the relaxation period, but also it will prevent you from demonstrating a good massage – your mind won't be on the job in hand!

Conduct massages for the same baby in the same place where possible so that the baby associates this with massage and pleasure. Low noise level is required; try using a gentle piece of music. If the same piece of music is used each time the baby will begin to recognise 'massage time'. It goes without saying that the area you are using should be clean and tidy, but also hygienic.

Once the room and area being used is prepared it is time to prepare the carer. The treatment should be explained and, where required, questions answered.

**SAFE PRACTICE**

*Remember always get the carer's consent before you begin to demonstrate massage. Unfortunately in today's society it is all too easy to be accused of criminal conduct: babies are vulnerable and should be protected at all times, but it means you must remember to protect yourself from any possible accusations.*

# Massage Mediums

A massage medium is a product that is used to help with 'slip and glide' in massage. Whatever medium you use, it is advisable to apply via the hands rather than pouring directly onto the skin as this gives the masseur the opportunity to warm both the oil and their hands prior to commencement of the massage.

**SAFE PRACTICE**

*It is advisable to patch-test a baby's skin, at least half an hour before treatment to make sure they are not allergic to it. Take a little oil and place it on the elbow crease of the baby's arm. This can be administered up to 24 hours prior to the massage, but if it is done before preparation begins and the consultation starts, then you will usually see a reaction within 20 minutes. If the test is positive, the skin will look pink to red and will irritate the baby. In such a case, use calamine lotion to soothe the irritation. If there is no reaction on the skin then it is safe to proceed with the treatment.*

The following mediums can be used:

## Vegetable Oils

These nourish the skin and have a pleasant feel. With babies it is wise to use an oil that is as natural as possible to avoid skin reaction. In particular nut oils should be avoided. Unrefined oils are preferable, for example, virgin olive oil.

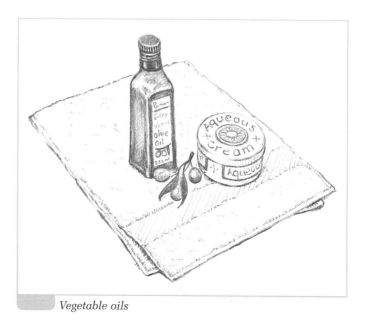
*Vegetable oils*

## The Advantages of Vegetable Oils

Natural plant oils can have a dramatic effect on the skin. Applying oils directly to the skin provides it with many of the nutrients needed to keep it supple and strong. Skin needs a rich supply of vitamins and essential fatty acids to keep it in good condition, all of which are found in vegetable oils.

Vegetable oils are especially rich in:

**Vitamin E** – This vitamin is often referred to as the 'vitality vitamin' because of its repairing and regenerating properties. It is an anti-oxidant which means it is able to neutralise **free radicals**, which cause cell damage.

Free radicals are a normal by-product of the body's metabolism, but in excess they are undesirable. They destroy **collagen** and **elastin fibres** that support the skin and they also interfere with the formation of fresh, new skin cells making complexions blotchy and dull.

**Vitamin A** – This aids in the replenishing of skin tissue. Vitamin A controls the rate at which skin cells are replaced. Lack of this vitamin leads to slow cell renewal, resulting in sallow, scaly complexions.

**Vitamin D** – This vitamin helps to promote healing and affects the quality and tone of the skin.

**Lecithin** – This nutrient is found in all vegetable oils and is an important component of cell membranes.

**Essential Fatty Acids** – These are necessary for building the membranes that surround every living cell, and play an important part in preventing moisture loss from the skin's surface. They can therefore assist in the delay of the onset of the ageing process. Examples are **linoleic** and **gamma linolenic acid (GLA)**.

The best vegetable oils to use are olive oil or grapeseed oil, which has a lighter texture. However, olive oil is the most nutritious.

---

**SAFE PRACTICE**

*Mineral oils are a by-product of petroleum and are not recommended for use as a massage medium. There are various 'baby oils' on the market which are often used on sensitive skins as the molecules of these oils are too large for absorption and therefore are unlikely to cause an allergic reaction. However, they do not have nutritional value for the skin, and they form a film on the skin that is not absorbed, which:*

- *does not allow the skin to breathe. Over long-term use makes the skin dry*
- *leaves the babies skin too slippery for safe handling if excess is not wiped off after massage*
- *can be ingested by the baby when it puts its hands (or even feet!) into its mouth.*

---

## Creams

These are not so easy to massage with as they are not so readily absorbed by the skin and tend to 'dry up' quickly. However, they are useful if a baby does not respond well to oil. Aqueous cream can be used as it contains no perfume or additives – it is easily obtained from a pharmacist and is inexpensive to buy!

For babies with eczema, cream is a good alternative, as the parent probably has to apply it regularly anyway.

### Lotions

Baby lotion can used, but it is even more quickly absorbed than cream. This means you would have to use large quantities, and it is also difficult to warm in the hands prior to use.

---

**SAFE PRACTICE**

- *Do not use oils derived from nuts, i.e. almond, hazelnut or peanut. Some babies can have allergic reactions to the use of oils, and anaphylactic fits can be life-threatening.*
- *Do not use aromatherapy oils, these can be highly dangerous.*
- *Do not use talcum powder, as there is a danger of babies inhaling it. It is also claimed to be linked with cancer.*

---

# Getting Ready to Massage

Before commencing a massage, the practitioner and carer should prepare themselves. It is easy to forget that even though giving a massage is pleasurable it is also fairly hard work if it is to be performed correctly. Wearing comfortable clothing, removing shoes and warming the hands are just a few things of the things you can do to support yourself.

## Hand mobility exercises

Hand mobility exercises will give you relaxed, supple and mobile hands, which aids your massage technique. Have a go at the following exercises:

1 Make a fist, clenching and stretching the fingers quickly.

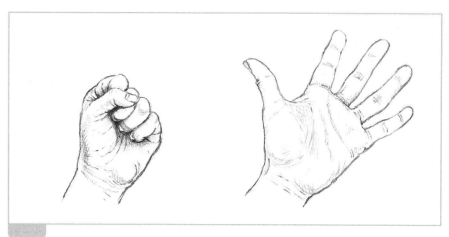

2️⃣ Roll the thumbs around, first one way, then the other.

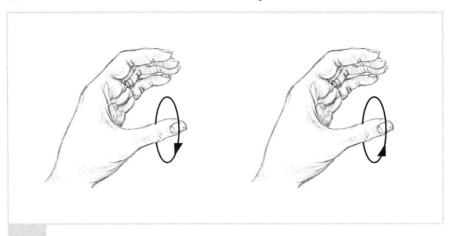

3️⃣ Roll each finger around, first one way, then the other.

4️⃣ Press the fingers back from the palms of the hands to their fullest limit.

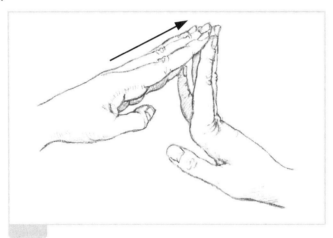

5️⃣ Place hands in a prayer position in front of the chest. Whilst maintaining contact press the hands downwards so that you can feel this action on the wrists and lower arm muscles.

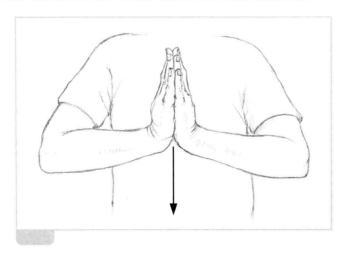

6 With the backs of the hands together, interlock the fingers and with the wrists apart try to pull the fingers apart.

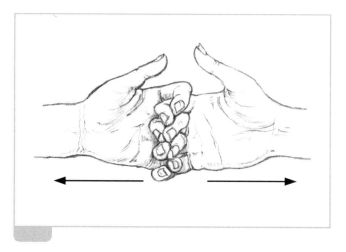

7 Make piano movements on a hard surface; try to maintain an even rhythm and aim to increase the speed.

8 Bend each finger back separately as far as it will go.

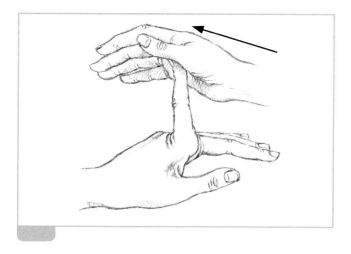

9 Finally shake the hands out.

## Breathing exercise

Now check your own and the carer's breathing rhythm to assess your general state of relaxation. If you are tense a baby will sense it and become tense. Breathe properly from your stomach: on inhalation, relax your stomach and let it expand with your chest. On exhalation blow out slowly and fully until the lungs are completely empty. Take several deep breaths to aid your relaxation.

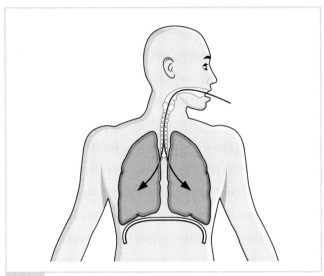

*Inhale, filling the lungs with air*

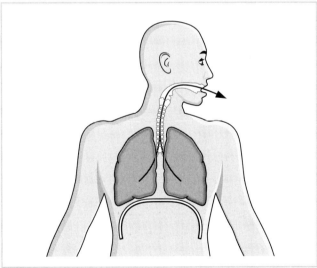

*Exhale slowly to enable relaxation*

Choose the position for the massage, either on the floor or the carer's lap. Ensure that the carer is relaxed and comfortable, otherwise the baby will sense this and become agitated.

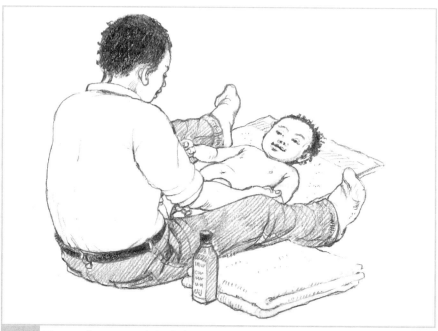

*Ensure that you and the baby are comfortable*

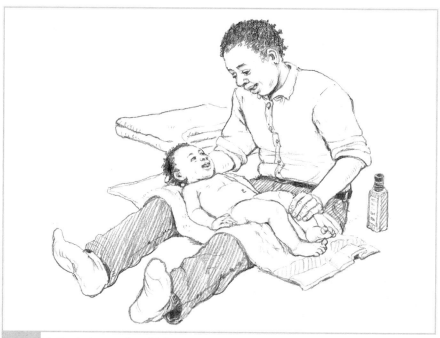

*Is the baby comfortable?*

As mentioned before, wear loose clothing, something comfortable that you don't mind getting oily, but remember you are a professional, keep it smart as well. Remove your shoes before you begin.

# Preparing a Baby

All babies are different – some more nervous than others, some more irritable – and so how you prepare a baby for massage will be pre-determined by the baby. Babies who are new to massage may respond more positively if you keep their clothes on for their first massage, building their confidence in the treatment. If a baby is happy to be undressed, massage them naked on a soft, warm, dry towel.

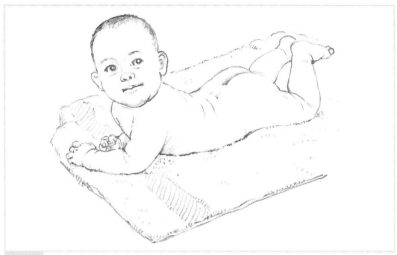

*Massage a baby without clothes only if they are comfortable with it*

Small babies up to four weeks old, do not usually like being undressed, so start by massaging gently over their clothes and then perhaps a vest until they are happy to be fully undressed. Never massage against a baby's wishes.

Remember to remove the nappy as this will definitely interfere with the routine. It is also much less restricting for babies – they love the freedom to kick their legs. Be prepared for them to urinate during the massage, this is a normal response – in particular watch out for little boys!

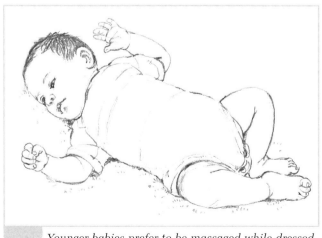

*Younger babies prefer to be massaged while dressed*

## REFRESH YOUR KNOWLEDGE

1. Why would you perform a patch test before commencing a massage?

2. Name two massage mediums you can use and one you cannot use.

3. What is the benefit of using a vegetable oil?

*for answers, see page 134*

# Your practice notes

# Performing the Massage

## The Classification of Massage Movements

Massage is the manual manipulation of body tissue. There are four main groups which can be sub-divided according to their function and effect on the body tissues.

1. Effleurage (Stroking):
   - superficial
   - deep
2. Petrissage (Kneading or Compression):
   - kneading (palmar, thumb, digital)
   - wringing
   - rolling
   - picking up
3. Tapotement (percussion): do not use on babies.
   - hacking
   - cupping (very gentle cupping on fleshy areas can be used on babies)
   - pounding
   - beating
4. Vibrations (Shaking): do not use on babies.
5. Frictions: do not use on babies.

### Effleurage

Effleurage is derived from the French 'effleurer' meaning to 'skim over'. It is a stroking movement. Hands can be used alternately, both together or just one. On smaller areas the finger tips can be used rather than the whole palmar surface. The pressure may vary from deep to superficial.

### Superficial Effleurage

This is performed with extremely light, even pressure, using the entire palmar surface of the hands. The fingers are held together. Massage always begins and ends with this movement. The pressure is so light that it does not affect the main circulation.

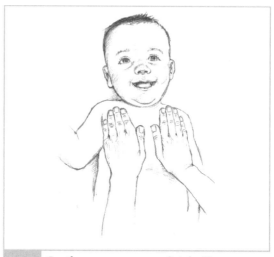

*Gentle pressure – superficial effleurage*

**The benefits and effects of superficial effleurage:**

- introduces a masseur's hands to a baby and aids the application of the massage medium
- is used as a linking movement between other movements and to get from one area of the body to another
- sedates and relaxes
- aids skin circulation and has a soothing effect on sensory nerve endings in the skin.

## Deep Effleurage

Any effleurage that is given with significant pressure is termed deep effleurage. The pressure may vary from moderately deep to very deep, but the pressure chosen should remain constant, otherwise tissues can be bruised, particularly on small areas. Pressure must always be directed towards the heart to assist the venous and lymphatic return.

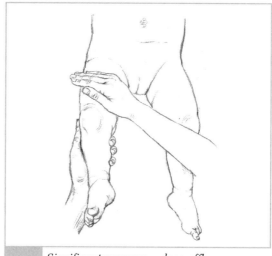

*Significant pressure – deep effleurage*

**The benefits and effects of deep effleurage:**

- aids venous circulation and indirectly aids arterial circulation by relieving congestion in the veins. Aids nourishment and oxygen to cells
- aids lymphatic circulation, hastening the removal of waste products
- relaxes tense and tight muscles
- aids capillary circulation in the skin, and the input of nutrition into the skin's tissues, improving elasticity and suppleness
- aids desquamation (skin shedding) and skin texture.

## *Petrissage*

Petrissage is derived from the French word 'pétrir'– to knead. It is also known as 'kneading' or 'compression'. It means compression movement performed using intermittent pressure, either with one hand, both hands or part of the hands. It consists of grasping or compressing a muscle group, a muscle or part of a muscle, and applying pressure, then releasing the pressure, progressing to an adjacent area and repeating the process. The technique involves lifting the tissues away from underlying structures, i.e. bone. The movement often follows the shape of the muscles, working from their insertion to their origin. Kneading movements are often described by the part of the hand used to accomplish the massage, i.e. palmar or thumb kneading.

Petrissage or kneading incorporates varying manipulations, such as:

- palmar kneading
- finger/digital kneading
- thumb kneading
- picking up
- wringing
- skin rolling.

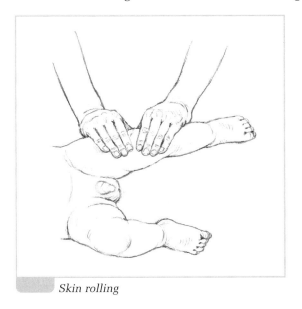

*Skin rolling*

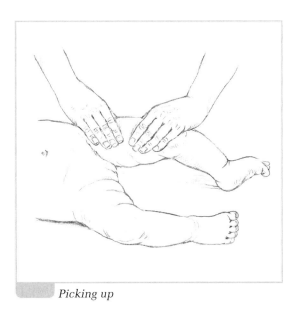

*Picking up*

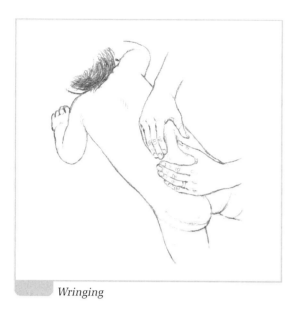

*Wringing*

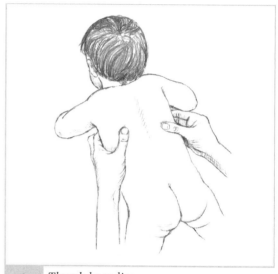

*Thumb kneading*

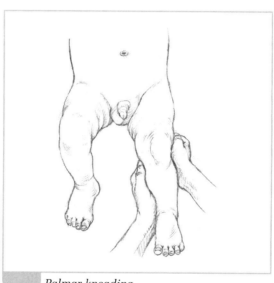

*Palmar kneading*

**Pressure** – Although the pressure is intermittent, great care must be taken to avoid pinching the skin and superficial tissues. To avoid this the pressure should be gradually reduced as the bulk of the tissues diminishes under the hand. The pressure used must vary according to the purpose of the massage and the bulk of tissues under treatment.

**Direction** – This depends on the purpose for which the massage is being given. For example: when massaging a limb, the massage may be started proximally, with each succeeding movement performed more distally, providing the heavy pressure is applied centrally to aid venous and lymphatic flow.

to have the baby in a comfortable, relaxed position

to perform the movements slowly, gently and rhythmically

to make the part of the hand used conform to the contour of the area under treatment

to use effleurage freely to link the petrissage movements in a purposeful manner

it is very important to ensure that movements are executed with relaxed and supple hands.

**The benefits and effects of petrissage:**

- The compression and relaxation of muscle tissue causes veins and lymph nodes or vessels to be filled and emptied, thus increasing their circulation and the removal of waste products.
- Fresh nutrients are encouraged into the tissues, thereby nourishing and feeding them.
- By increasing the deep muscular circulation, lactic acid is removed, so eliminating fatigue and pain.
- The skin – both superficial and deeper tissues – are all stimulated to further activity.
- Correctly applied compression produces a toning effect on muscular tissue which can act as a reinforcement to natural exercise.
- Skin rolling is especially effective on **adipose tissue**.

Note: Petrissage is more effective in aiding the absorption of substances within tissues, than is deep effleurage.

Deep, purposeful petrissage serves to squeeze lymph from the lymph spaces. Followed by deep, centrally applied effleurage, the lymph is moved to the nearest group of lymphatic nodes which aids in efficient drainage and helps in the removal of excess fluid, i.e. **oedema**.

reflect

Working in pairs, practise deep and superficial effleurage and petrissage on each other's arms, closing your eyes when you do this. Use this opportunity to practise both your technique and the pressure you administer.

Now evaluate: how did it feel, did the pressure change, were you conscious of the movement that was being done?

## REFRESH YOUR KNOWLEDGE

1 Which massage movements can be safely used in baby massage?

2 What is the effect of petrissage?

3 In which direction should you always massage?

*for answers, see page 134*

# Introductory Massage Routine for Premature and Newborn Babies

## Premature Babies

Premature babies are incubated and have very little touch from humans. The only touch they do receive is often negative, in the form of injection tubes being administered, etc. They therefore associate touch only with pain and become very nervous when eventually they are able to be held.

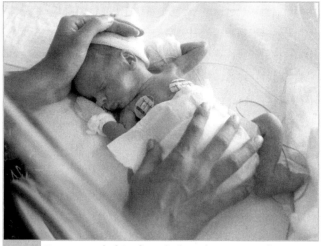

*Premature babies benefit from human touch*

Research into massage and the premature baby in the 1980s provided evidence supporting the fact that the grasp and suckling reflex, which is very poor in premature babies, is greatly improved if they are able to have massage. It means babies move onto oral feeding and from ventilator to cot more quickly. Their general immunity is improved so they can go home more quickly, and they grow far more rapidly than their control counterparts.

Some hospitals readily accept massage and touching premature babies, but others do not; it all depends on the consultant in charge. Advise the parents/carer to ask permission and explain why they feel the need for this method to be applied to a particular baby. Most doctors will agree if the baby is not too seriously ill.

Research shows that touching stimulates peripheral and autonomic nervous systems, so reducing the need for monitors and supports. Place warm hands on accessible parts of the baby's body. Maintain the contact daily, as often as possible, gradually increasing the duration of touching. When holding becomes possible, hold the baby close to you, just stroking with warm relaxed hands. Then, when you are able to introduce a light massage, keep the baby clothed and follow the introductory routine.

Once you are able to, massage with oil, as premature babies have very dry skin. When babies are pre-term, they are more vulnerable than full-term babies, so do not insist that they straighten their limbs, which remain folded for longer for self-protection.

## Babies up to 4 Weeks

Newborn babies do not like to be undressed as it makes them feel insecure. Start by massaging the baby through their clothes. When they seem to have got used to this, undress them and, providing they like to be naked, follow the introductory routine, but remember not to massage the chest or abdomen as the lungs and stomach are still sensitive after birth.

**SAFE PRACTICE**

*Newborn babies have difficulty keeping warm during the first month of their lives and should be kept at a room temperature of around 20 degrees centigrade, day and night. So it is important that a baby is warm for their massage.*

# Your practice notes

# The Introductory Massage Routine

## SAFE PRACTICE

*Remember to warm up the oil by standing the bottle in a bowl of hot water, kept well out of the way of the baby, for a few minutes, so that it is up to hand temperature. Test on the inside of your wrist before applying! Make sure your hands are warm, too!*

The following routine is not meant to be prescriptive and should be adapted to suit the individual child or baby. Some children will prefer to be stroked, while others may need to placed in a different position – take your cue from the child.

Position yourself comfortably and so that you will be undisturbed for at least half an hour. Turn on some soothing music and dim the lights – now you are ready to begin. Lie the baby on their side next to you and facing you. Gently stroke down their side from the top of the shoulder to the foot covering the arm, side, hip, leg and foot. The baby should find this soothing and relaxing. Do this for one minute (see below).

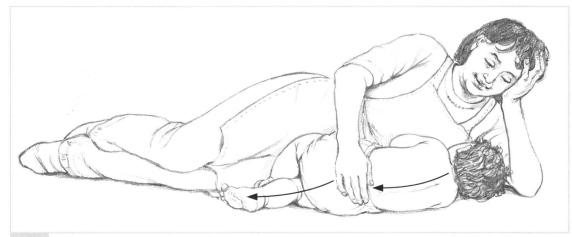

*Gently stroke from the top of the shoulder to the foot*

Next, in the same position, gently circle the whole of your hand in a clockwise movement up and down the baby's back and over the buttocks, making sure the circles are large and the rhythm slow, for two minutes.

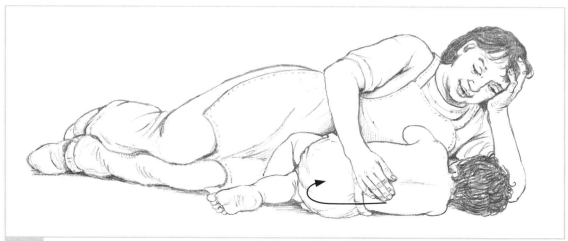

*Use a clockwise, sweeping movement over the baby's lower back and buttocks*

Now massage the baby's lower back and over their buttocks in a sweeping movement clockwise, again for two minutes. Now repeat these movements on the other side of their body (see above).

If the baby will lie happily on their front, stroke your hand down their back from the shoulders to the base of the spine for about a minute with each hand (see below).

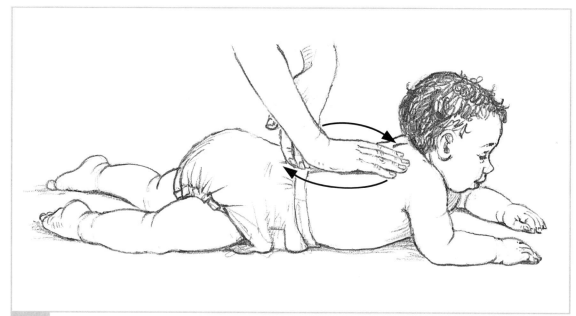

*Use alternate hands to stroke up and down the baby's back*

Once the baby has become used to this introductory routine, which should last about ten minutes, you can move on to the full baby massage routine next time.

# The Baby Massage Routine (Four Weeks and Onwards)

Once the baby is used to a light introductory massage and they are happy to be undressed, the full massage routine can be used.

## Timing

The massage can be performed at any time of the day when the baby feels comfortable, not too tired or hungry. A good time is mid-morning, half an hour after the baby has digested their feed and before their morning sleep. Then hopefully the baby will remain much calmer for the rest of the day. At night, after the bedtime bath is probably the most preferable and beneficial time as it relaxes the baby for sleep.

On average, the massage takes a good half an hour but it could be as short as ten minutes if the baby does not relax. It will vary each time, but take the initiative from the baby; the massage length should be in accordance with the baby's tolerance. If they are enjoying it then perhaps massage for a little longer; if not, then shorten the routine. As with adult massage, there can be no set time.

## REFRESH YOUR KNOWLEDGE

1. What temperature should be maintained for newborn babies?

2. How would you go about preparing the oil ready for use?

3. Why do we sometimes start by massaging a fully clothed baby?

4. When is it a 'good time' to massage a baby?

5. When is it not desirable to massage a baby?

*for answers, see page 135*

# The Baby
# Massage Routine

Before you start, have you remembered to:

✓ warm the oil

✓ wash your hands

✓ take the phone off the hook

✓ put on any music you plan to use (if you are using music)?

The following routine is a guide from which the practitioner can base his or her treatment. The practitioner can differentiate each routine as appropriate i.e. in the same way that some people do not enjoy having their feet being massaged, so might the child or baby – remember always let the child or baby's cues to guide the massage.

The more of the routine that is completed the more effective the treatment will be, however it is not essential to complete each routine. For each area of the body start with an effleurage movement, build up to a deeper massage using petrissage, and then finish with an effleurage movement again.

With the baby on their back begin by stroking them from head to toe.

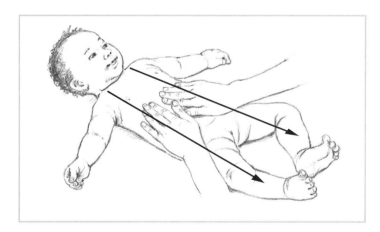

**1 Effleurage** – with the baby's foot sandwiched between the palms of your hands, gently, but firmly, effleurage the length of the foot keeping the toes stretched. Do this several times, particularly if the foot feels cold to the touch.

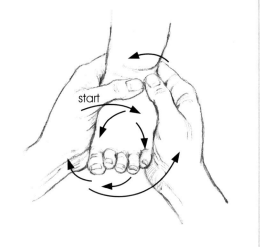

**2 Friction** – rub the feet between your hands, backwards and forwards.

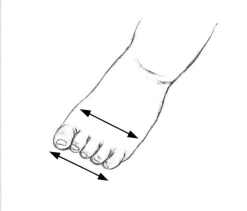

**3 Circles** – with fingertips placed each side of the ankle, make small circles towards you, clockwise.

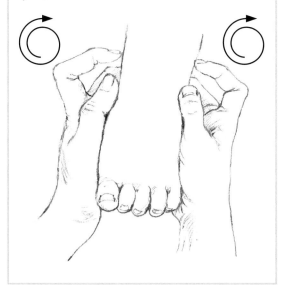

**4 Stroking** – spread the toes and stroke the top of the foot several times to finish.

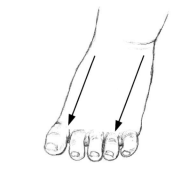

**1** **Indian milking** – starting with one leg, draw your hands down the leg firmly, hand-over-hand to the foot. Do this several times, then repeat the movement on the other leg.

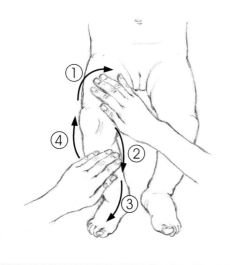

**2** **Rolling** – roll the leg between your palms and thumbs starting at the top of the thigh, then working down to the toes, moving the hands alternately in a circular motion. Do this several times, then repeat the movement on the other leg.

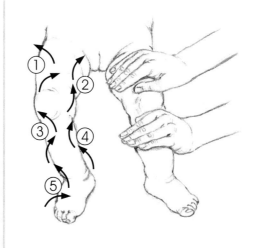

**3** **Squeezing and twisting** – with your hands underneath the thigh and thumbs on top, squeeze the thigh gently whilst pulling your thumbs apart, then bring them back together again. Making a twisting movement, move down the whole leg to the foot and then back up to the thigh. Do this several times, then repeat the movement on the other leg.

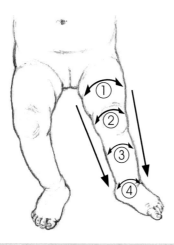

**4** **Stretching** – working on both legs, place your thumbs on the inside of the thighs, fingers on the outside, and gently pull down around the thigh, then down the back of the knee, calf and finally the feet. As the baby straightens their legs, give a very gentle stretch when you get to the feet.

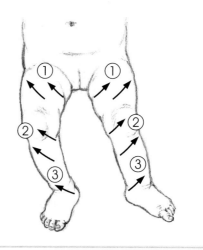

**5** **Bicycling** – holding gently onto the baby's feet, pedal the legs three or four times then clap the soles of the feet together playfully.

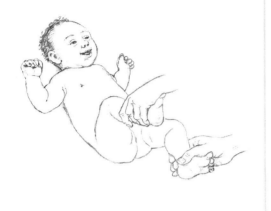

**6** **Swedish milking** – working on one leg at a time, gently squeeze, working up the leg, one hand over the other to the thigh.

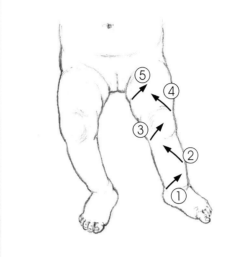

**7** **Stroking** – finish the leg massage by gently stroking down both legs.

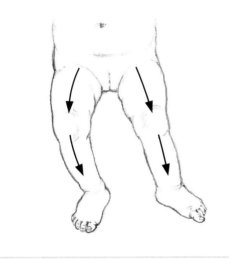

Confident babies stretch out their arms during a massage; less confident or nervous babies tend to pull their arms in towards the centre of their bodies, and some babies won't allow massage of their arms at all. Remember, never force a massage on a baby; be guided by his needs and desires.

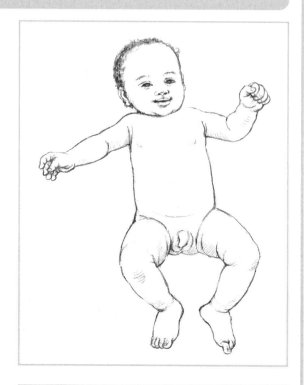

**1** **Stroking** – working both shoulders together, stroke from the top of the shoulder to the finger tips. Repeat this several times.

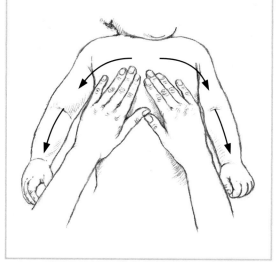

**2** **Indian milking** – starting with one arm, draw your hands down the arm firmly, hand-over-hand to the fingers. Do this several times, then repeat the movement on the other arm.

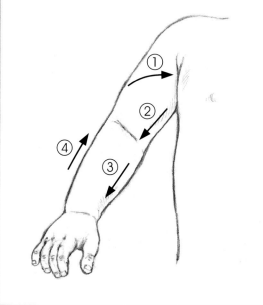

**3** **Rolling** – roll the arm between your palms and thumbs down the arm towards the fingers, moving the hands alternately in a circular motion. Do this several times, then repeat the movement on the other arm.

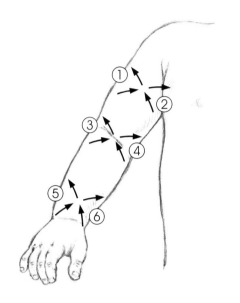

**4** **Squeezing** – gently squeeze up the arm to the shoulder, one hand over the other. Do this several times, then repeat the movement on the other arm.

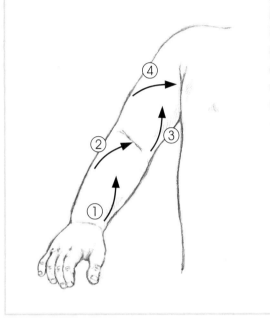

**5** **Stroking** – complete the arms by gently stroking both of them together from the top of the shoulders to the fingertips. Repeat several times.

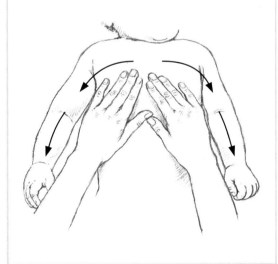

**1** **Stroking** – with your hands flat, and gently resting on the baby's chest, stroke upwards and outwards towards the arms, keeping the palmar surface in contact with the baby, but without firm pressure.

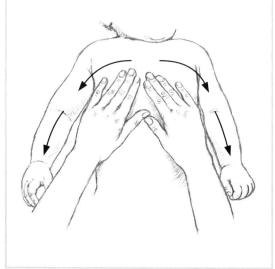

**2** **Prayer** – with your hands in the centre of the chest, over the sternum, and together as if in prayer, open them out in a gentle gliding motion, sliding to the shoulders and down the arms to the fingertips. Repeat several times.

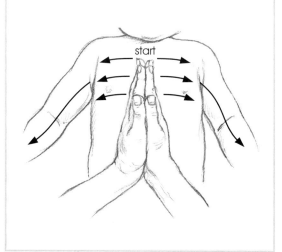

**3** **Cross stroking** – using your hands alternately with a stroking movement, work from the lower to the upper chest, crossing over to opposite shoulders.

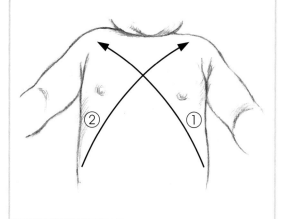

**4** **Thumb stroking** – with your thumbs together and facing upwards, pull apart across the nipple line. Repeat several times.

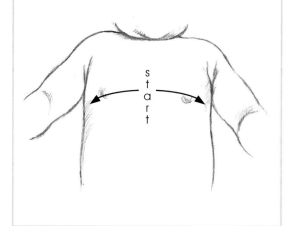

**⑤ Stroking** – repeat the first movement (see above).

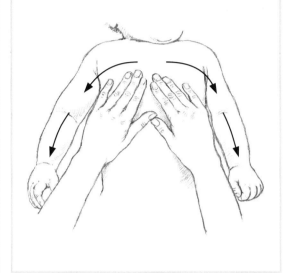

**⑥ Clapping** – clap the baby's hands together playfully, unless they object.

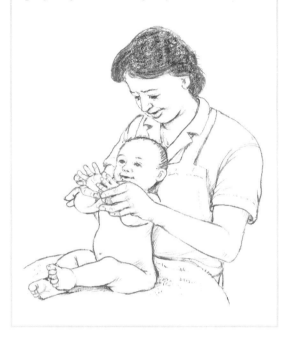

**⑦ Armpit circles** – this is a very sensitive area, so great care must be taken to use only light pressure. Move your thumbs in a gentle circular motion, working just in front of the armpits. Repeat this two or three times only.

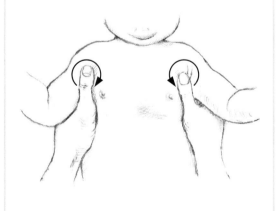

**⑧ Stroking** – repeat the first (and fifth) movement (see above), two or three times.

**1** **Turning wheel** – with one hand after the other, and working from left to right, using the palm of the hand, stroke with the motion of a turning wheel. Repeat two or three times.

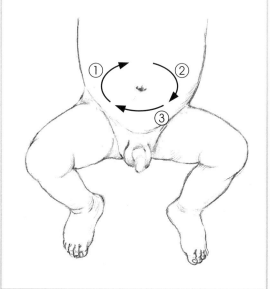

**2** **Flat strokes** – with your left hand flat across the abdomen and your right hand above facing the opposite direction, change the position of the hands so that as the top hand moves down, the bottom hand moves over it to the top position. Repeat several times.

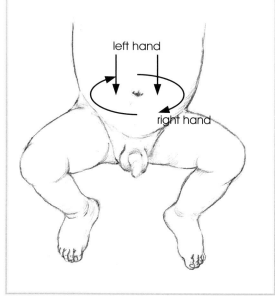

left hand

right hand

**3** **Fingertip stroking** – with the baby in front of you, using your fingertips, and starting on your left, stroke the abdomen up to the rib cage, across and then down the other side. Repeat two or three times.

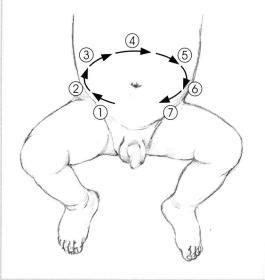

4 **Side stroking** – gently stroking the baby's sides, draw your hands upwards and inwards. Repeat on both sides.

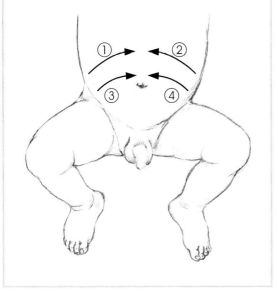

5 **Sweeping** – place the heal of your hand just above the pubis bone, with fingers spread, and sweep across from left to right without removing the heel of your hand. Repeat two or three times. Use gentle pressure for this movement as too much pressure will cause discomfort, especially on the bladder area.

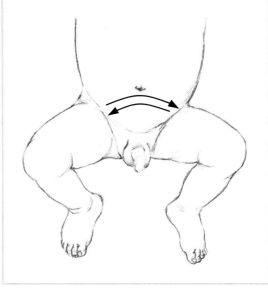

**1** **Thumb stroking, forehead** – using either your thumbs or fingertips, smooth out from the centre of the forehead to the edge of the forehead. Repeat two or three times.

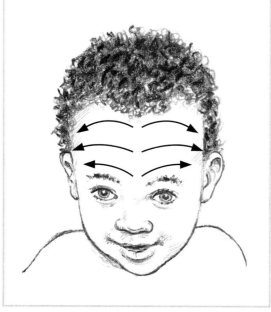

**2** **Fingertip stroking, eyes** – with light feathery movements and middle fingertip, work from the bridge of the nose around the eyes two or three times.

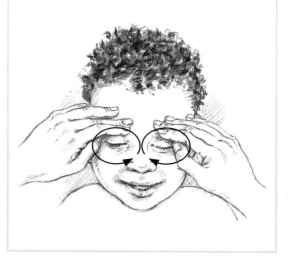

**3** **Fingertip stroking, nose** – gently stroke from the bridge of the nose down to the corners of the mouth two or three times.

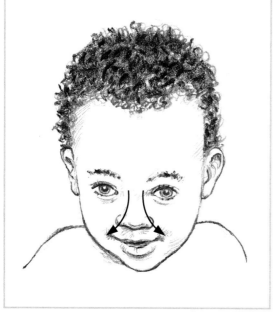

**4** **Fingertip stroking, mouth** – using the same finger, starting under the nose, circle around the mouth to meet on the chin, two or three times.

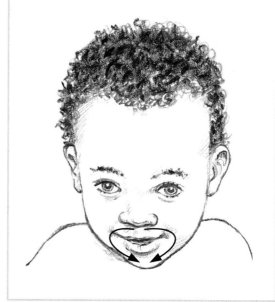

**5** **Fingertip stroking, jaw line** – starting at the point of the chin, work out towards the ears along the jaw line. Repeat several times.

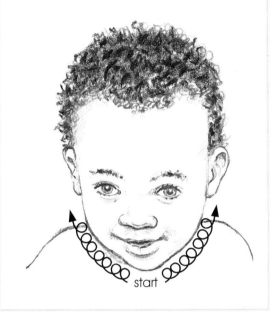

start

**6** **Ears** – with your index finger, massage around the ears, finishing with a gentle pull on the lobes.

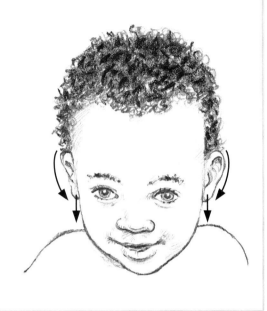

**7** **Whole head** – using the whole palm of your hand, and working with alternate hands, stroke up and over the forehead, over and down the back of the head to the bottom of the neck, six times.

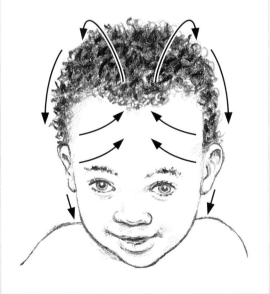

Finish the front of the body with gentle stroking from head to toe, repeating a few times.

**1** **Stroking** – begin by stroking from the neck to the lower back using both hands alternately. Repeat a few times.

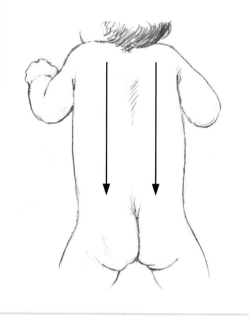

**2** **Palmar shuffling** – move the palms of your hands backwards and forwards up and down the whole of the back several times.

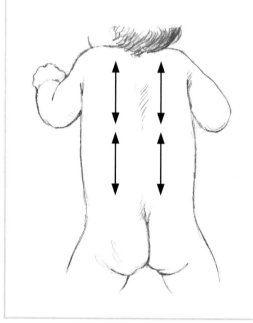

**3** **Spine circles** – with hands either side of the spine, starting at the base, work up and down the length making small circles. Repeat several times.

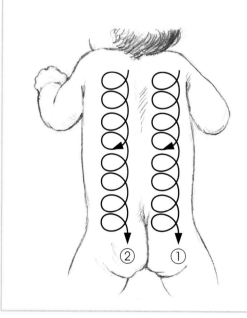

**4** **Spine stroking** – very gently, but not so as to tickle, stroke downwards from the spine several times using your fingertips and alternate hands. Do not stroke directly over the spine.

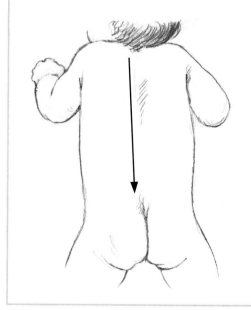

**⑤ Cupping** – cup your hands, place either side of the spine, and without force gently pat down the back from top to bottom. Repeat two or three times. Do not use cupping over the child's shoulder as this may be uncomfortable.

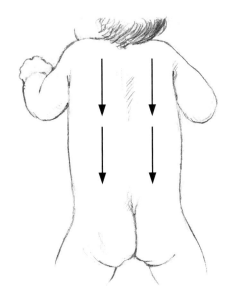

**⑥ Cat's paws** – finish with gentle full stroking down the spine using the full palm of your hands in an alternate movement.

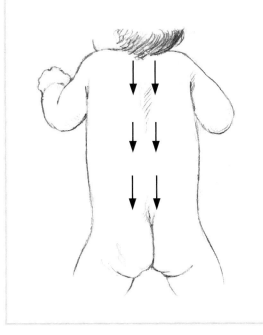

# BUTTOCKS

**1** **Encompassing** – with both of your hands together at the base of the spine, slide apart, outwards and then downwards, up and back together, encompassing the buttocks and repeating several times.

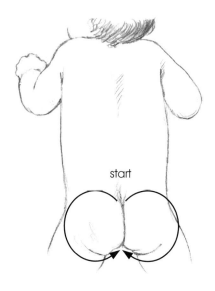

start

**2** **Kneading** – gently knead the buttocks by massaging around the base of the spine (not on it), and into the fatty tissue with relaxed hands.

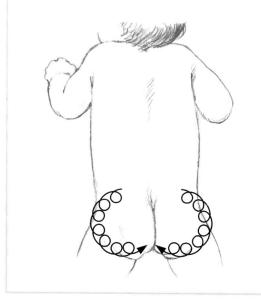

**3** **Stroking** – finish by stroking the whole of the back, around the buttocks and back to the top of the spine. Repeat three or four times.

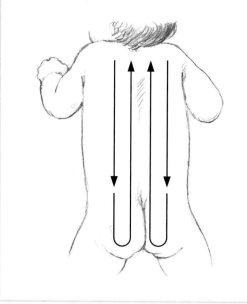

Wrap the baby up in a towel and give them a cuddle; he or she is probably hungry now!

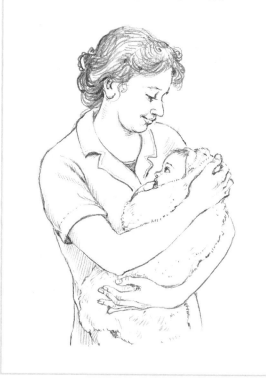

# After-care

All babies react differently to massage – some feel sleepy, while others are invigorated and often hungry – therefore it is difficult to give after-care advice other than to follow a baby's lead! Clearly, if a baby doesn't enjoy the massage and appears fractious afterwards, then the advice would be to discontinue the treatment. However, this rarely happens – in fact, more often the advice would be to continue massaging as frequently as every day. For babies who feel tired it would be best to perform the massage before bed, and for those who become invigorated, to massage mid-morning.

- If vegetable oil has been used let it remain on the skin for at least one hour so that it can nourish the skin.
- If a mineral oil has been used, or any oil in excess, blot the skin before applying nappy and clothes.
- Allow babies to rest for at least half an hour after massage. They will probably be hungry – so feed them!

If massage is to be given before bedtime, then bath the baby first. The warmth of the bath and the massage will relax them and open the pores to allow greater absorption of the oil, and they should sleep well!

# Your practice notes

# Evaluating the Massage

A formal evaluation should always be carried out and recorded at the end of a baby massage, and there should be a space for this on your evaluation sheet (see page 127–8). There are several observations that should be made.

## Effectiveness of the Massage

The effectiveness of a massage will depend on many factors: how confident and relaxed the baby was when you started, the atmosphere, the bonding between parent/carer and child, the confidence with which the baby was handled, and many others. To determine if a massage has been effective you must look for several changes. These are detailed below:

- **The skin** – has it changed colour; is it blotchy, very pink or glowing? Skin reacts to massage, every baby being different depending on the sensitivity of the skin, the colour to begin with, and how warm the baby was.

- **Temperature** – the temperature of a baby should remain the same as it was before you started the massage. Although you are increasing the circulation through massage, you are also increasing elimination, therefore the body continues to stabilise the temperature both before, during and after the massage. However, the temperature of the skin should feel warm to the touch as a direct result of massage.

- **Temperament** – not all babies respond well to massage; in fact some won't let you near them! But, for those who do, it is usually a soothing, calming experience for the baby which will be reflected in their temperament. Babies are often thirsty or hungry following a massage treatment, so if you find a baby fractious give them a bottle before making a note about their temperament! You should note a baby's reactions both during and after a massage: how alert they were, were they sleepy, happy or unhappy, etc.

- **Joint mobility** – babies are usually very flexible without massage, but giving a series of treatments over a period of time improves a baby's joint mobility. Ensure that you record any increase in movement/the suppleness of the baby.

- **Bonding** – before you can ascertain an improvement you first need to be aware of the current state. Before you start a massage, watch the relationship between parent and child. Parents who are uncomfortable with touching and being close may become tense every time a child reaches for them. Conversely a 'touchy, feely' parent will feel confident with their child, and in turn the child with them. This will become more easily recognisable with experience.

## REFRESH YOUR KNOWLEDGE

1. Explain how you would evaluate the effectiveness of the massage.

2. What does it mean if a baby's skin turns pink and blotchy after a massage?

3. Name the after-care points the practitioner should give at the end of the massage.

*for answers. see page 135*

# Your practice notes

# PART THREE:
## Experiencing Massage

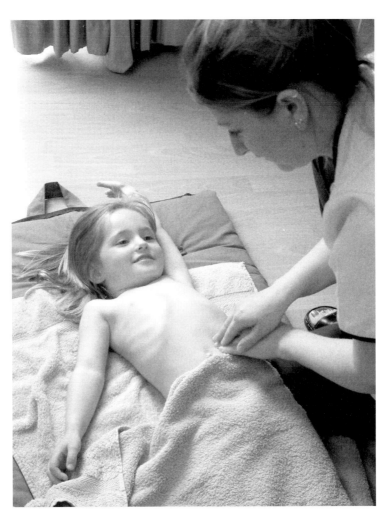

# Group Demonstrations

There are a variety of settings you might choose: the local health centre, a hospital, a hall, someone's house, a school, a playgroup or a college – the list is almost endless. Before doing anything else you need to plan your demonstration: who are you going to demonstrate to, where, when and how long is it going to take, what will you need and how do you prepare? On the surface it seems comparatively easy, but in reality it takes a lot of organising. This chapter is aimed at helping you to answer all of these questions. Follow these steps to simplify the task.

- Start by thinking about all the groups of people that you could demonstrate to, for example a group of mums at a clinic or a group of midwives in a hospital.

- Who do you know? Think about all your connections, friends who are parents, friends of friends, etc., then make a list and start asking around; once you have one carer you will be led to others. There won't be many of you who really don't have a connection somewhere; you need only one person to get the ball rolling. You may be looking to teach mothers: one mum will agree to come along, and before you know it you will have them arriving so fast you will have to start turning people away!

- Once you have identified your group you will need to introduce yourselves. You may want to get help constructing a letter introducing yourself and announcing the demonstration, or you may want to visit your local health centre and give a talk to the local health visitor and a group of mums. A 'drop-in' clinic is a good way to get to know people; go along with a handout explaining a bit about yourself and the demonstration you want to do, chat with people while they are waiting, then sign them up!

- Set the date and begin the preparations. Check how many people are going to attend – between six and eight is preferable (too many and you won't cope, too few and you won't have a group)!

- Instruct each person in your group to bring a baby's changing mat, a large towel, a change of clothes and a bottle of milk.

- You will need some gentle music, oil and cream, a large 'baby-size' doll and a roll of kitchen paper (just in case!) and your paperwork.

- The paperwork should consist of a handout for clients to take away, which should contain contra-indications, do's and don'ts, the routine and aftercare. If you have access to an overhead projector, it would be advisable to put your routine onto acetate, leaving you free to help the carers. You will need a feedback sheet for them to complete at the end of the demonstration, which will be used as evidence towards your qualification.

- Choose a venue that is airy but warm, clean, and has toilet and washing facilities.

- On the day of the demonstration arrive at least 15 minutes early. This will give you time to get set up before anyone arrives.

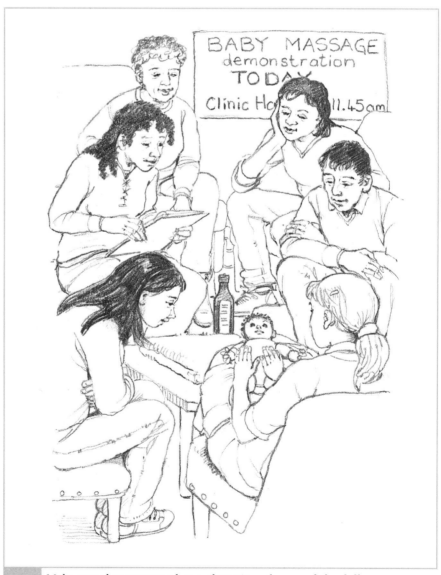

*Make sure that everyone has a clear view of you and the doll*

- Once your carers arrive, get them to sit round on the floor in a large semi-circle, with you at the front so that they can see you, and you can see them!
- Check all the babies for contra-indications, check the carers have removed their jewellery and explain how the session is going to take place.
- Get the carers to set up, and when everyone is ready you can begin your demonstration – good luck!
- At the end of the demonstration answer any questions the carers may have and ask them to complete the feedback sheet. Make sure that you complete all the record cards and evaluations before the carers leave.

**SAFE PRACTICE**

*Remember, if you are working with more than one baby, you will be running a risk of cross-infection. It is essential that you do not go from one baby to another without first washing your hands. Towels and changing mats should not be shared and carers must be encouraged to touch only their own babies.*

*Prior to the demonstration it is a good idea to ask carers not to attend if either they or their baby is feeling unwell, as even a simple cold will be easily spread in a warm room.*

# Example of a Group Demonstration Questionnaire

Carer's name ..................................................

Please take a few minutes to answer the following questions and add any comments you feel may be helpful to improve the demonstration.

| | | |
|---|---|---|
| 1 | Did you find the demonstration interesting? | Yes/No |
| 2 | Had you heard of baby massage before today? | Yes/No |
| 3 | If yes to question 2, please state where. | Yes/No |
| 4 | Have you ever massaged your baby before today? | Yes/No |
| 5 | Would you like to continue to learn more massage movements? | Yes/No |
| 6 | Did you understand the benefits of massage? | Yes/No |
| 7 | Do you feel encouraged to massage your baby at home? | Yes/No |
| 8 | Did your baby enjoy the massage? | Yes/No |
| 9 | Does your baby's skin look healthier? | Yes/No |

Please use this space to add any comments you feel would be useful:

# Your practice notes

# Case Studies

Some of the following case studies will be similar to your own experiences, others are remarkable; all of them however are true accounts. The babies' names have been changed to protect their identity.

## CASE STUDY

*Danny was your regular, average baby, if there is such a thing! 7lb 8oz at birth, breast-fed, no complications, sleeping reasonably well, happy and alert, nine weeks old – but motherless. Danny was living with his grandmother who had devoted all her time to him for the last three weeks and had pledged to for the rest of her life.*

*When Grandma phoned a massage practitioner, she explained that she felt there was a 'bond' missing between her and Danny, something that she could not replace from the loss of his mother, her daughter. However, she wanted to try to bring Danny and herself closer, to increase his feeling of security with her, and the health visitor had recommended massage as a way forward.*

*Danny responded brilliantly, he loved his massage, and so did Grandma. They both responded straight away, Danny confidently allowing Grandma to massage his arms away from his body and Grandma concentrating hard on learning the routine.*

*The practitioner visited the house only three times, but in that time could clearly see how both were enjoying the pleasure of massage and the closeness that it can bring. It is at times like that when you can see all of that hard work and training is worth while!*

## reflect

In groups, discuss Danny's case study and consider all the psychological aspects relating to both the grandmother and Danny. Why do you think the health visitor recommended baby massage? How do you think something so simple could fill such a large void in both Grandma and Danny's life?

*Hayden* *was ten weeks premature, weighing in at 2lb 12oz. His lungs collapsed at birth, which resulted in a long stay in hospital for both him and Mum. Eight months later he was brought to a massage practitioner. The consultation revealed the everyday picture that is so often missed by the 'onlooker': it seemed that most of the time Hayden was fractious, woke several times a night, was prescribed steroids for psoriasis and wouldn't drink from a bottle – exhausting!*

*Mum and the practitioner set to work, starting with a gentle massage and leaving Hayden's clothes on for this first treatment. Hayden enjoyed his front being massaged, but wasn't so keen on his back being done, so they cut short the routine and finished with a gentle rocking in Mum's arms.*

*The practitioner's visits were planned daily and for the same time – just after bath and before bed. By the third visit they had Hayden stripped off and volunteering to lie down for them in anticipation!*

*Upon returning for the fourth visit, Mum came running to the gate to greet the practitioner. 'Last night he slept, all the way through, he didn't wake up, I can't believe it!' she exclaimed. 'It's the massage, it must be, and I have noticed today he's not so fractious, in fact this is the happiest I have seen him!'*

*Hard to believe, but the massage really had had the effect Hayden's mum had described; she continued to massage Hayden every day, at the same time in the same place with the same music. Hayden learnt to relax and enjoy this time, learning very quickly that massage meant sleep time – and so he did.*

reflect

1 What would you do if Hayden hadn't enjoyed his first massage?

2 Do you think Hayden would have benefited by having the massage earlier in his life?

3 What would have been the benefits, and at what stage would you have massaged him?

*Suzie*, *a healthy 9lb 12oz at birth, enjoyed her first massage at three months old, fully clothed and lying in Mum's arms. As you would expect with any young baby, Suzie slept for short bursts, ate, filled her nappy and then resumed the cycle so familiar to so many of us!*

*For the second massage the practitioner decided to formalise the massage routine. Dad chose music that he felt comfortable with while Mum bathed Suzie and wrapped her in a warm towel in preparation for her first 'real' massage. Mum had found the massage uncomfortable, and so they agreed that this was to be Dad's moment, a part of his daily routine shared with his daughter. Dad had a lot to learn! His hands were rough, and his movements jerky, unnerving Suzie who became upset very quickly.*

*The practitioner decided that if this was to succeed, then Dad needed to be taught the art of massage before he started practising on his daughter again. He was also booked in for a manicure with paraffin wax immediately!*

*The practitioner called round the next day, only this time the practitioner took a large doll with her. Dad was clearly not sure about this, but instead of giving him time to think, the practitioner prepped up and got on with the business of teaching him how to massage without pulling the legs off!*

*After a week of leaving Dad to get on with it and practise, the practitioner returned. Clearly this was a very determined man who was not going to be beaten by either his daughter, or a doll! Dad had worked extremely hard and had learnt the routine, practising every evening until he had perfected the routine.*

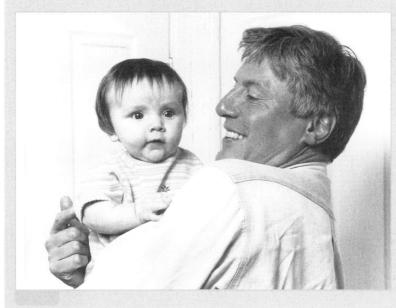

*Suzie enjoyed the massage. She was confident, allowing her arms to be stretched out to the side and her legs to be mobilised.*

*The success of this story was not so much in the impact the massage had physiologically, but the way in which it brought father and daughter a new dimension to their relationship.*

reflect

1. Would you have pushed Suzie's mother harder to get her more involved in the massage?

2. What impact do you think this would have had on the 'family'?

*Charlotte was a gentle, shy baby, who clung to Mum for dear life when she saw the practitioner coming! She was ten months old, with no previous experience of being massaged. Given this, the practitioner decided the best way to introduce the massage was on an 'informal basis'. Sitting opposite one another, both in armchairs, the adults chatted about Charlotte while the practitioner completed the record card. A handy tip when visiting slightly older babies at home for the first time is to take your own baby with you – not a real one of course! A large doll, Charlie, sat on the practitioner's lap during the consultation, whilst Charlotte sat on her mother's lap. Instructing Mum to follow the lead and copy everything that was done with Charlie, the practitioner began by holding Charlie in her arms, facing the doll which lay on its side, gently stroking from the top of its head to the tip of its toes. Charlotte wasn't having any of it; she knew the practitioner was in the room and desperately wanted to keep her eye on her!*

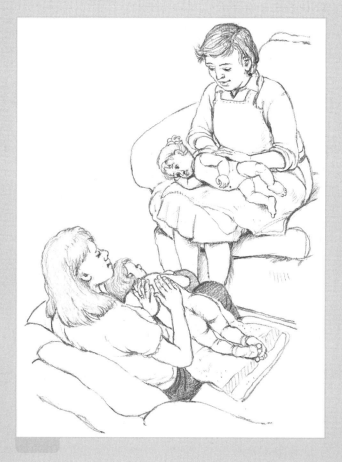

*So the practitioner turned Charlie over onto the other side facing Charlotte, and Mum did the same. That was better: Charlotte could see everything that was going on. The practitioner ignored her, all*

*bar a quick smile or two, and continued to massage Charlie. When they could see Charlotte beginning to relax the practitioner took Charlie's hand and began palmar kneading, Mum following, Charlotte watching!*

*Finally, after five minutes, it was too much and Charlotte had had enough. The practitioner suggested that Mum continued to do the same movements just before bed that same night, only this time to both sides and both hands, if Charlotte would allow it.*

*The practitioner returned the next day and they attempted the same routine. A little over five minutes passed and again Charlotte decided enough was enough!*

*It took nine attempts to get Charlotte to settle in for eight minutes of massage. Mum and the practitioner decided that she was not the sort of baby was ever going to allow more than this. However, they did both agree that it was good quality time with each other and that the benefit of mother and daughter being close in this way at the end of the day was worth the nine visits the practitioner had made.*

## reflect

1. What other technique could have been used to relax Charlotte?

2. Do you think the result would have been different if the massage routines had been started earlier in Charlotte's life? If you do, then in what way could it have been different?

3. Why do you think children like Charlotte don't enjoy massage?

*Violet, a baby massage practitioner, had a client whose child's left foot had been amputated as a result of a car accident. When Violet noticed that child's foot was missing she told the child's carer that she thought it best not to massage the left leg at all as it would not be possible to complete the whole routine. Violet completed the treatment, instructing the carer to avoid the left leg – she even suggested that the carer avoid massaging the right leg so that the child would not feel 'unbalanced'.*

*Violet later admitted to another colleague, Simon, that she was 'repulsed' by the amputation and was scared to massage the amputated area. Simon assured her that it was safe, in fact very beneficial, for the child to be massaged and that is was important that Violet respond in a professional and caring way and ask the child's carer to include the both legs in the next massage treatment.*

## reflect

1. It is difficult for you to gage just how you might respond to a baby or child with an amputation, how do you think you could prepare yourself beforehand?

2. How do you think Violet should have responded in this situation?

3. In what ways do you think massage could help both the child and her carer?

# Your practice notes

# PART FOUR:
## Supporting qualification documentation

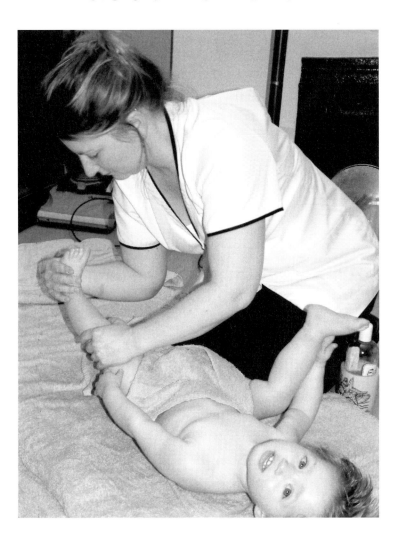

The following forms are the supporting qualification documentation that will help you gain the most out of your qualification. They have been designed in a way that will allow you to photocopy the blank versions of the forms, so that you can fill them out and keep them as a record of your work.

# Baby massage consultation form

Ref. Number .............. S6 ..................................................... Date ./.July.2003...

| Baby's first name | James | | Mothers details | |
|---|---|---|---|---|
| Date of birth and Age | 12.12.02 | 7 months | Name | Avril |
| Sex | Male ✓ | Female | Date of birth | 01/04/62 |
| Weight at birth | 3.8 kg | | Number of children | 1 |
| Current weight | 9.5 kg | | Medical | Post natal depression |
| Physical abnormalities | None | | | |
| Medical history (Illness, diseases, disorders, operations, allergies) | Medication/immunisation<br>All immunisations up to date. Normal birth, no infections, no known allergies to date. | | | |
| Contra-indications | None | | | |
| Sleeping habits | Sleeps for three hours at a time, wakes constantly during the night. During the day sleeps twice, mid-morning and mid-afternoon | | | |

| Personality | Happy | Fractious | Both | Comments |
|---|---|---|---|---|
| | | ✓ | | Mum thinks it is because of the broken sleep |

**Parent/Guardian declaration:**

I declare that the information I have given about my baby is true and correct as far as I am aware. He/she can undertake treatment with the practitioner without any adverse affects. I have been fully informed about contra-indications and treatment guidelines and limitations and therefore I am willing for the practitioner to proceed.

Parent's signature .........*Avril Smith*................... Date ../.July.2003...

# Baby massage consultation form

Ref. Number ................................................................. Date ......................

| Baby's first name | | | Mothers details | |
|---|---|---|---|---|
| Date of birth and Age | | | Name | |
| Sex | Male | Female | Date of birth | |
| Weight at birth | | | Number of children | |
| Current weight | | | Medical | |
| Physical abnormalities | | | | |
| Medical history (Illness, diseases, disorders, operations, allergies) | Medication/immunisation | | | |
| Contra-indications | | | | |
| Sleeping habits | | | | |

| Personality | Happy | Fractious | Both | Comments |
|---|---|---|---|---|
| | | | | |

**Parent/Guardian declaration.**

I declare that the information I have given about my baby is true and correct as far as I am aware. He/she can undertake treatment with the practitioner without any adverse affects. I have been fully informed about contra-indications and treatment guidelines and limitations and therefore I am willing for the practitioner to proceed.

Parent's signature ...................................................... Date ......................

# Baby massage treatment and evaluation sheet

Baby's first name and ref. number ...... James S6 ...... Date .... 1. July 2003 ....

Parent/Guardian first name ................ Avril ................ Treatment number .one..

| Massage movements used | ✓/✗ | Areas massaged | ✓/✗ | | ✓/✗ | Massage medium used | Detail |
|---|---|---|---|---|---|---|---|
| Effleurage | ✓ | Face | ✓ | Back | ✓ | Cream | |
| Petrissage | ✓ | Abdomen | ✓ | Head | ✓ | Oil | Olive oil |
| Stretching | ✓ | Arms | ✓ | | | Other | |
| Joint manipulation | ✓ | Legs | ✓ | | | | |

## Timing of treatment

Full massage completed, 50 minutes total

## How parent coped with massage; any problems

Mum did really well, had some prior massage experience so teaching the techniques was not difficult. She found it hard working on such small areas like the arms and feet in particular

## Evaluation of treatment

## Physical and physiological responses of baby (i.e. skin condition, colour, texture, joint mobility

Skin colour pinked up as we worked, texture was dry to begin with but feels softer now, joint mobility was excellent to begin with. James felt warm at the end of the treatment but not too hot.

## Psychological response of baby (i.e. general disposition before, during and after treatment, interaction of parent and baby).

James interacted well with mum, eye contact was good throughout, was slightly fractious during the facial routine but settled well, seems tired now but defiantly more relaxed.

Parent's comments, signature and treatment evaluation:

Really enjoyed the time James and I spent together learning the massage

*Avril Smith*

Therapist's comments and evaluation:

James and his mum clearly enjoyed the massage, they worked well together. The oil has made a huge difference to James skin, it was very dry to begin with. Mum has requested the next treatment involves Dad – appointment booked for 4.7.03

# Baby massage treatment and evaluation sheet

Baby's first name and ref. number ............................ Date ...........................

Parent/Guardian first name ....................................... Treatment number ........

| Massage movements used | ✓/✗ | Areas massaged | ✓/✗ | | ✓/✗ | Massage medium used | Detail |
|---|---|---|---|---|---|---|---|
| Effleurage | | Face | | Back | | Cream | |
| Petrissage | | Abdomen | | Head | | Oil | |
| Stretching | | Arms | | | | Other | |
| Joint manipulation | | Legs | | | | | |

**Timing of treatment**

**How parent coped with massage; any problems**

**Evaluation of treatment**

**Physical and physiological responses of baby** (i.e. skin condition, colour, texture, joint mobility

**Psychological response of baby** (i.e. general disposition before, during and after treatment, interaction of parent and baby).

Parent's comments, signature and treatment evaluation:

Therapist's comments and evaluation:

# Treatment log

**Candidate's name** ........................... **Candidate number** .........................

**Requirements for assessment:**
**Date:** the date the treatment is given
**Portfolio ref. no.:** Page number in portfolio
**Baby ref. no.:** unique reference number given to baby at time of consultation
**Baby range:** to include nervous/non-nervous, irritable, age, new & existing
**Treatment range to include:**
- used cream/oil/lotion
- demonstration to individuals or to groups
- areas massaged.

| Date | Portfolio ref. no. | Baby ref. no. | Baby range | Treatment range |
|------|--------------------|---------------|------------|-----------------|
|      |                    |               |            |                 |
|      |                    |               |            |                 |
|      |                    |               |            |                 |
|      |                    |               |            |                 |
|      |                    |               |            |                 |
|      |                    |               |            |                 |
|      |                    |               |            |                 |
|      |                    |               |            |                 |

| Date | Portfolio ref. no. | Baby ref. no. | Baby range | Treatment range |
|---|---|---|---|---|
| | | | | |
| | | | | |
| | | | | |
| | | | | |
| | | | | |
| | | | | |
| | | | | |
| | | | | |
| | | | | |
| | | | | |
| | | | | |
| | | | | |

# Baby Massage Theory Assessment

1. What legislation and codes of practice are concerned with standards of hygiene in premises used for massage?

2. Name four contra-indications to massage.

3. What action would you take if you establish a baby has a contra-indication at the consultation/preparation stage?

4. List two psychological benefits of baby massage for babies.

5. List three benefits to the parents/or carer.

6. Name the massage supports you can use and one you cannot use.

7. Name two massage mediums you can use and one you cannot use.

8. What is the benefit of using a vegetable oil?

9. Describe the type of movement called effleurage?

10. Which massage movements can be used on a baby and which cannot be used?

11. Give two ways in which massage could benefit premature babies.

12. How would you maintain client confidentiality when filling in the consultation form?

13. How long should you wait before massaging a baby after a vaccination?

14. Give three after-care instructions.

*for answers, see page 135–7*

# Baby Anatomy and Physiology Assessment

1. What is the first fluid excreted from the breast before breast milk?

2. What is the function of this fluid?

3. What is a baby's first stool called?

4. Why is sterile powder (or talcum powder) no longer used to aid healing of the umbilical cord?

5. What substance is a baby's skin covered with a birth?

6. Name two functions of this substance.

7. What are the effects of massage on the abdominal organs?

8. In which direction should the colon be massaged?

9. What is ossification?

10. Name the five reflexes with which a baby is born.

*for answers, see page 135–8*

# Answers

## Answers to Refresh your knowledge: page 15

1 The Local Government (Miscellaneous Provisions) Act 1982.
2 Practitioners should always portray a professional image. A client may assume that a 'scruffy' practitioner lacks care for his or her profession and will therefore perform a 'scruffy' treatment.
3 The Health & Safety at Work Act 1974.
4 Any three of the following:

| THE EMPLOYER IS RESPONSIBLE FOR: | THE EMPLOYEE IS RESPONSIBLE FOR: |
| --- | --- |
| ensuring the premises is safe, with access to exits | ensuring he or she avoids personal injury |
| systems and equipment | assisting the employee in meeting the health & safety requirements |
| storage & transport of substances & materials | avoiding injury or danger to clients |
| good practices | not misusing or altering anything that has been provided for safety. |
| distributing information on health & safety to employees | |
| ensuring there is adequate ventilation, correct working temperature, appropriate lighting, client privacy & low noise levels | |
| protecting employees from heath & safety risks. | |

5 See page 14 for reference.

## Answers to Refresh your knowledge: page 29

1 The five reflexes are suckling & swallowing, rooting, grasping, walking and startle.
2 Any two of the following:
   - is able to reach and grab items
   - passes toys from one hand to the other
   - makes a variety of sounds
   - is able to focus fully as eyes work together now
   - laughs and chuckles with delight when he gets attention.

3 Having a good understanding of a child's development age will support your professionalism, enable you to identify a child's developmental age and will give you confidence to work with babies and children.

## Answers to Refresh your knowledge: page 48

1 A baby's lungs are collapsed in the uterus as they have not yet been inflated and oxygenated. The baby absorbs oxygen via the placenta which is then carried through its circulatory system.
2 Foramen ovale and the Ductus Arterosus.
3 The babies clotting power at birth is low because newborn babies are often low in Vitamin K. Vitamin K is needed by the liver for the production of Prothrombin, one of the elements necessary for clotting blood.
4 Brown fat is used as fuel to supply heat and also acts as an insulating layer for the baby.

## Answers to Refresh your knowledge: page 72

1 A patch test is performed prior to massage to ensure that the baby or child does not have any sensitivities or an allergic reaction to the medium being used.

2

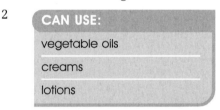
**CAN USE:**
vegetable oils
creams
lotions

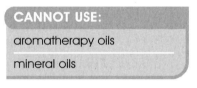
**CANNOT USE:**
aromatherapy oils
mineral oils

3 Vegetable oils are natural plant oils providing the skin with a rich supply of nutrients, vitamins and fatty acids, which are easily absorbed into the skin.

## Answers to Refresh your knowledge: page 80

1 Massage movements that can be safely used on baby are effleurage and petrissage.
2 The effects of petrissage are:
  ● increased waste removal
  ● increased nourishment to the tissues
  ● lactic acid is removed thus eliminating fatigue and pain
  ● fibrosis is prevented via the relaxation of contracted muscles
  ● skin renewal is stimulated
  ● muscles are toned which re-enforces natural exercise
3 You should always massage towards the heart.

## Answers to Refresh your knowledge: page 85

1 Room temperature should be kept around 20° centigrade day and night for newborn babies.

2 Oil should be warmed prior to use – place a small bowl of oil into a larger bowl of boiled water.

3 Newborn babies in particular do not like to be undressed, it makes them feel insecure and cold.

4 Massage is recommended before the baby goes to bed, after a bath or prior to his or her mid-day sleep.

5 A baby should never be massaged when he has just eaten, when he is hungry or asleep.

## Answers to Refresh your knowledge: page 104

1 The effectiveness of a massage can be determined by looking at the following factors:
- skin change
- temperature
- temperament
- joint mobility
- increased bonding.

2 Skin sensitivity will differ between babies, the more blotchy and pink it is the more sensitive the child's skin is, and indicates that the skin has been well stimulated.

3 Any of the following:
- if vegetable oil is used it should remain on the skin for at least one hour so that it can nourish the skin
- allow the baby to rest for at least half an hour following the massage
- if the baby is hungry, feed him!

## Answers to Baby massage theory assessment: page 131

1 The Local Government (Miscellaneous Provisions) Act 1982, and Professional Code of Practice for Beauty Therapists, Care workers and Health practitioners.

2 Contra-indications are any of the following:
- if the baby is asleep
- *has been recently immunised
- has a skin disorder or infections
- is hungry
- has had recent surgery

- is currently undergoing treatment for a medical condition and GP approval has not been given
- has a dysfunction of the nervous system
- has had a recent haemorrhage
- *swellings, cuts bruises or abrasions
- *recent fractures or sprains.

NB Some of these contra-indications are localised to areas of the body and are indicated by *.

3 If a contra-indication has been discovered then the massage should not proceed unless it is minor and a local contra-indication, such as swellings, cuts bruises or abrasions or has been recently immunised.

4 The psychological benefits of baby massage include:
- a strengthening in bond between carer and child
- feeling of well-being.

5 Benefits to the parents or carer include:
- involving the whole family
- strengthensing the relationship and bonding between parent (particularly male) carers and child

6

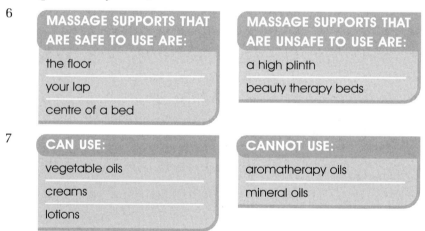

| MASSAGE SUPPORTS THAT ARE SAFE TO USE ARE: | MASSAGE SUPPORTS THAT ARE UNSAFE TO USE ARE: |
|---|---|
| the floor | a high plinth |
| your lap | beauty therapy beds |
| centre of a bed | |

7

| CAN USE: | CANNOT USE: |
|---|---|
| vegetable oils | aromatherapy oils |
| creams | mineral oils |
| lotions | |

8 Vegetable oils are natural plant oils providing the skin with a rich supply of nutrients, vitamins and fatty acids which are easily absorbed into the skin.

9 Effleurage is a stroking movement that is used to link movements, and to start and end a massage routine. There are two types, the first is a superficial movement that is performed with extremely light, even pressure. The second is deep effleurage and is performed with significantly increased pressure and effects the underlying tissues and central circulatory system.

10

| MASSAGE MOVEMENTS THAT CAN BE USED ON BABY ARE: | MASSAGE MOVEMENTS THAT SHOULD NOT BE USED ARE: |
|---|---|
| effleurage | tapotment |
| petrissage | friction |
| | vibrations |

11  Massage can benefit premature babies by:

- improving their grasping and suckling reflexes, moving them onto oral feeding quicker
- immunity is improved, enabling them to leave hospital more quickly
- touching stimulates the peripheral and autonomic nervous systems, reducing the need for monitors and support.

12  There are a number of different systems that can be adopted to protect client confidentiality. Try to use coding or reference numbers, and not names, on the client record cards and keep references separate from the client cards. It must be remembered that everything a client tells you is in the strictest of confidence and should not be discussed except with the client themselves.

13  Before massaging after immunisation ensure that the area is no longer sensitive, the redness and any swelling should no longer be visible.

15  After-care advice, any of the following:

- if vegetable oil is used it should remain on the skin for at least one hour so that it can nourish the skin
- allow the baby to rest for at least half an hour following the massage
- if the baby is hungry, feed him!

## Answers to Baby anatomy & physiology assessment: page 132

1  Colostrum.

2  Colostrum provides the baby with a high level of protein that contains less fat and sugars than milk and aids in the production of globulins and immunoglobulins which are absorbed by the body. The most important of these is the immunoglobulin IgA which provides the defence against bacteria and viruses in the bowel.

3  Meconium.

4  Talcum powder is a component of sterile powder and research has linked it to cancer.

5   Vernix Caseosa covers the baby at birth.

6   Vernix Caseosa acts as a lubricant during birth, protects the skin and helps to retain heat.

7   Massage to the abdominal organs can help to relieve constipation and colic.

8   The colon should be massaged clockwise, i.e. from left to right which naturally follows the route of the alimentary tract.

9   Ossification is the process whereby cartilage develops into bone.

10  The five reflexes are suckling & swallowing, rooting, grasping, walking and startle.

# Qualification Cross-referencing

## Contents

| Contents | Ref. for Baby Massage Certificate | Ref. for Level 3 Teaching Cert in Baby Mass. | Page no. |
|---|---|---|---|
| Introduction/The history of massage | U.K. | U.K. | 1–3 |
| Professional ethics/code of practice | El1 – R1 | El1–R2 E.K. El1 | 7–9 |
| Legislation | El1 – R1/R2/R3 | El1–R1 E.K. El1/El 2 | 9–13 |
| Maintaining employment standards for the therapist | El1 – R2 | El1–R3 E.K. El1 | 13–5 |
| Stages in the growth and development of a child | U.K. | | 17–31 |
| Related anatomy and physiology | E.K. El 3 | | 37–48 |
| The growth of the skeleton | E.K. El 3 | | 37 |
| The blood | E.K. El 3 | | 38 |
| The effects of massage on the muscular system | E.K. El 3 | | 39 |
| Foetal circulation/respiration | E.K. El 3 | | 40–1 |
| The effects of massage on the lungs | E.K. El 3 | | 41 |
| The lymphatic system | E.K. El 3 | | 42 |
| The effects of massage on the nervous system | E.K. El 3 | | 44 |
| The skin | E.K. El 3 | | 45 |
| The digestive system | E.K. El 3 | | 46–7 |
| Colostrum | E.K. El 3 | | 46 |
| The function of the liver | E.K. El 3 | | 46 |
| The urinary system | E.K. El 3 | | 47 |
| Contra-indications to baby massage | El2 – R2 | El2–R2 | 51–2 |
| Hygienic baby massage treatment | El2 – R1 | | 61 |
| Massage support | El2 – R3 | El2–R3 | 62 |
| Preparation for massage | U.K. | El2–R1/R3/R4 | 62 |
| Massage mediums | El3 – R4 El2–R2 | El1–R5 | 63 |
| Getting ready to massage | U.K. | | 66 |
| Preparing a baby | El2 – R4 | E | 71 |
| The classification of massage movements | El3 – R5 | | 75 |
| The introductory massage routine for premature and newborn babies | E.K. El 2 | | 80 |
| Premature babies | U.K. | | 80–1 |
| The baby massage routine (four weeks and onwards) | El1 – R5 | | 83–100 |
| After-care | El4 – R4 | El3–R2/El 4–R1/R4 | 101 |
| Evaluating the massage | El4 – R1,R3, R4 | El1–R4/El 4–R1/R4 | 103–4 |
| Group demonstrations | El3 – R3 | El2–R1 E.K. El2 El3–R3 | 109–12 |
| Case studies | U.K. | El2–R4/El3 | 115–20 |
| Baby massage theory assessment | E.K. El1, 2 & 3 | | 131 |
| Baby anatomy and physiology assessment | E.K. El3 | | 132 |
| Babies with special needs | E.K. 4–El4 | El2–R4 | 53–6 |
| How babies communicate | E.K. 4–El4 | | 31–5 |

**KEY**: U.K. = Underpinning Knowledge; E.K. = Essential Knowledge; El = Element.

# Useful Addresses

**International Association of Infant Massage (IAIM)**
56 Sparsholt Road
Barking
Essex IG11 7YQ
Tel: 0208 5911399
Email: mail@iaim.org.uk
Web: www.iaim.org.uk

**The Guild of Infant and Child Massage (GICM)**
22 Elder Close
Uttoxeter
Staffs ST14 8UR
Tel: 07796 916 179
Email: mail@gicm.org.uk
Web: www.gicm.org.uk

**Federation of Holistic Therapists**
3$^{rd}$ Floor, Eastleigh House
Upper Market Street
Eastleigh
Hants SO 509 FD
Tel: 023 8 048 8900
Email: info@fht.org.uk
Web: www.fht.org.uk

**VTCT Customer Service Department**
Unit 11, Brickfield Trading Estate
Brickfield Lane
Chandlers Ford SO53 4DR

**Association for Spina Bifida and Hydrocephalus (ASBAH)**
42 Park Road
Peterborough PE1 2UQ
Tel.: 01733 555988
Web: www.asbah.org

**British Council of Disabled People**
Litchurch Plaza
Litchurch Lane
Derby DE24 8AA
Tel.: 01332 295551
Minicom: 01332 295581
Fax: 01332 295580
Web: www.bcodp.org.uk

**Cystic Fibrosis Trust**
11 London Road
Bromley BR1 1BY
Tel.: 020 8464 7211
Web: www.cftrust.org.uk

**Down's Syndrome Association**
155 Mitcham Road
London SW17 9PG
Tel.: 020 8682 4001
Fax: 020 8682 4012
Email: info@downs-syndrome.org.uk
Web: www.dsa-uk.com

# References and Further Reading

Kohner, N., Phillips. A. and Ford. K. (1994) *Birth to Five*, London: Health Education Authority

Meggitt, C. (2001) *Baby and Child Health,* Oxford: Heinemann

Staerker, Dr P. (2000) *Tender Touch: Massaging Your Baby to Health and Happiness*, Los Angeles: Price Stern Sloan.

Stoppard, Dr M. (2001) *Conception, Pregnancy & Birth: The Childbirth Bible for Today's Parents,* London: Dorling Kindersley

Tassoni, P. (2003) *Supporting Special Needs: Understanding Inclusion in the Early Years*, Oxford: Heinemann

Weston, T (1997) *Atlas of Anatomy*, Australia: Sandstone Publishing

# Index

**J**

joint mobility and strength 37

**K**

kneading 78, 100
 also see petrissage

**L**

lactic acid 39, 79
language 24, 26, 28, 31
legislation 9–13
 Children Act (1989) 12–3
 Data Protection Act (1998) 13
 Health and Safety at Work Act
  (1974) 11–2
 Local Government Act (1982) 10
 RIDDOR 12
limb loss 55, 120
Ling, Peter Henry 3
lung function and strength 41, 56
lymphatic system and massage 42,
 55, 56, 77, 78, 79

**M**

massage movements 75–9
medical ethics 9
mediums used in massage 63–6
milking 88, 89, 90
modes of expression 20
muscular system and massage 2,
 38–9, 55, 77, 79

**N**

needs 31
nervous system and massage 43–4,
 76, 81
newborn babies 2, 20, 42, 81

**P**

pain 1, 2, 20, 33, 44
peristalsis stimulation 47
personal protective equipment 11,
 13
petrissage 3, 42, 44, 75, 77–9, 86
 also see kneading
physical benefits 2
physical contact 1
physical health 1, 2
premature babies 2, 80–1, 116
preparation for massage 61–71, 86
professional development 8

professional ethics 7–8
protecting children, see legislation
psychological health 1, 2

**R**

record keeping 8
reflex actions 17–9, 80
refusal to massage 7
relationships 2, 20, 31, 104
relaxation 2, 69, 70, 76, 77, 79, 81,
 83, 85
reporting accidents, injuries,
 diseases 12
respect for individuals 7
respiration and massage 2, 41, 44
responsibility 7

**S**

safety checks 62
sense of security 55
sensitivity, tact and discretion 7
sensory impairments 53
skeleton and massage 2, 37
skin and massage 45, 76, 77, 79
skin disorders 9, 51
skin rolling 77, 79, 88, 91
skin shedding 45
soothing 1
special needs children and
 massage 53–6
speech, see language
spina bifida 56
standards of care 7
 see also hygiene; personal ethics
stroking 1, 58, 81, 83, 84, 86, 87,
 89, 90, 91, 92, 93, 94, 95, 96,
 97, 98, 100
 see also effleurage

**T**

tapotement 75
touch 1, 2, 22, 32, 80, 81, 104
toxin and waste product
 elimination 46, 47, 79

**V**

vegetable oils 63–5, 101
vibration 3, 75
visual impairment 54, 55

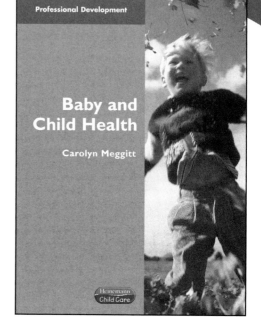